GET TOUGH!

The U.S. Special Forces Physical Conditioning Program

GET TOUGH!

The U.S. Special Forces Physical Conditioning Program

TOM FITZGERALD

St. Martin's Press / New York

Editor: Toni Lopopolo
Assistant Editor: Andrew Charron
Agent: Barbara Lowenstein

Library of Congress Cataloging in Publication Data

Fitzgerald, Tom.
  Get tough!

  1. United States. Army—Physical training.
2. United States. Army. Special Forces. 3. Exercises.
4. Physical fitness. I. United States. Army. Special
Forces. II. Title.
U323.F57   1985   613.7'1   85–11837
ISBN 0-312-32629-7 (pbk.)

First Edition

10 9 8 7 6 5 4 3 2 1

Illustration photographs by Gene Paltrineri, Dover, N.H.

for
Alan (Smoky) Sherman
1936–1984

It beat him—finally
Smoky
For it had to.
No cure, they said.
But it never defeated him.

There are still heroes among us.

Acknowledgments

I wish to express my deep appreciation to the United States Navy for their cooperation in the preparation of this book. A special thank you to Captain Thomas N. Tarbox.

I also wish to thank Dr. Edward Eldridge, Jr., for reviewing the manuscript, for his many suggestions and generosities, and for his genuine concern for athletes; Gene Paltrineri, for services above and beyond; Carol Rowe, Rodney Johnson, Matt Fitzgerald, and Bob Davis for volunteering themselves for the illustrations; Andy Charron and Toni Loppolo, for having the faith; and Jamie Brierton, for his continued friendship.

—Tom Fitzgerald

A Few Words from a Naval Special Warfare Officer

There is no "official" Naval Special Warfare physical fitness program. Each Underwater Demolition Team, SEAL Team, Swimmer Delivery Team, or Special Boat Unit has its own; and each of theirs varies somewhat according to the proclivities of the person or persons conducting it. However, all of these programs are based on the conditioning program developed, used, and revised in the same basic training the author of this book underwent to become a U.S. Navy frogman (officially, Basic Underwater Demolition/SEAL training, or BUD/S).

Needless to say, there have been significant changes to this program over the forty-two years since the first Underwater Demolition Teams were formed during World War II. To name just a few: the early prohibition against drinking water just before and during exercise has changed to hearty encouragement; and stretching exercises are no longer considered as just resting, but have become very important parts of the program. These and many other changes were initiated by advances in medicine and physiology, in coaching and athletic equipment, and by the general level of awareness facilitated by the media and public dissemination—but also by individuals such as Rudy Boesch, Bob "Doc" Clark, and Dan Rose, who were able to exert the right influence at the right time.

It is to be hoped that this book will also be one of those

right influences, but for a much wider audience. The program it describes is very similar to, and contains most of the "land" elements of (as you might expect, training in the water is also a rather important part) the Naval Special Warfare physical fitness program(s), but it is in a more comprehensive form.

We have used such a program for over four decades to ensure that our team members are *physically* capable of conducting whatever operations, including combat, are required of them. There is also, of course, mental conditioning, and skill and operational training, inherent in our basic and unit programs; but in order to make these effective, the individual frogman or SEAL must feel that, given the proper training, he is capable of doing anything required of him.

And he does—and you will feel the same about your strength and endurance when you complete the program presented in this book.

Because the body is exceptionally capable, much more so than even we think it is, when you complete the program presented in this book, you will: (1) feel very good about yourself, (2) want to stay with at least a modified version of it for the rest of your life, and (3) discover that a number of your other capabilities and potentials are also enhanced.

Take heed of Dr. Eldridge's advice on the following page, and also of the advice contained under the general instructions. I would say "Good luck," except that completing this program is not a matter of luck; it's a matter of how much you want the results.

—Thomas N. Tarbox

[Author's Note: A twenty-five-year veteran of the U.S. Navy, Captain Tarbox spent most of his career in Naval Special Warfare, for which he served tours as Director of Basic Underwater Demolition/SEAL training, and Commanding Officer of a SEAL team. The SEAL teams (SEa, Air, and Land) are among the U.S. military's most highly trained special forces units.]

A Few Words from a Doctor

With the plethora of physical fitness, running, and exercise books and magazines being published today, and the resultant "flooding" of the market, it is difficult to believe that anyone could produce a unique book on fitness. However amazing, Mr. Fitzgerald certainly seems to have accomplished that task. He has taken an intensive program of calisthenics and running, complemented it with a stretching program of proven worth, and presented it for the serious elite athlete or those who are capable, both physically and mentally, of attaining such stature in the world of physical fitness and conditioning. It is by no means intended for the sporadic weekend exerciser.

The stretching program provided is a major asset to the overall program. All too often athletes fail to realize the performance value of proper stretching. Although the time that must be invested in stretching is minimal, the benefit is enormous. A well-stretched, toned muscle is functionally superior to a tight one, and is also much less subject to injury. The stretching program presented herein is of the nonballistic type—the type considered best by most authorities today.

The U.S. Special Forces Physical Conditioning Program itself was designed to produce the uniquely high level of conditioning required by members of the U.S. Navy's elite frogman and SEAL teams. Members of these teams must perform physical and mental tasks on a daily basis that most of us would never encounter in a lifetime.

One word to the wise, as the saying goes. Because of the physical stress and intensity of this program, anyone contemplating participation should not do so without a thorough pre-participation evaluation by a medical practitioner of his or her choice.

Good luck in your quest for superior fitness!

—Edward E. Eldridge, Jr., M.D.

[Author's Note: Dr. Eldridge is the attending physician for the University of New Hampshire football and basketball teams.]

Contents

Contents

Tables

Introduction

The U.S. Special Forces Physical Conditioning Program is a challenging calisthenic and running program designed to condition the body to a superior level of physical fitness. It is based on the time-tested program used by the U.S. Navy to condition its famous frogmen and SEALS (SEa, Air, and Land), and is intended for anyone who is committed to enhancing his or her strength, agility, and endurance to the level of the competitive athlete.

No specialized equipment is necessary.

GET TOUGH!

The
U.S. Special Forces
Physical Conditioning
Program

The Program

The U.S. Special Forces Physical Conditioning Program consists of two separate programs that complement one another: the Calisthenics Program and the Running Program. These two programs run concurrently over a five-day week for twelve consecutive weeks, and are based on the theory of progressive development; that is, each program becomes increasingly more demanding with time—but gradually. The Calisthenic Program consists of a daily progression of calisthenic exercising directed at five different body areas. There are forty-six different calisthenic exercises, but you do not perform all forty-six on any one day. The Running Program consists of a daily progression of running with intermittent rapid walking; some of the running intervals include brief periods of sprinting.

Because this conditioning program aims to be a complete conditioning program, it includes a comprehensive stretching program. Designed for both before-workout stretching and after-workout stretching, the stretching program is based closely on the famous flexibility program developed at Penn State University and used by the Penn State football team.

Specific details concerning the Stretching, Calisthenic, and Running Programs follow a few important instructions.

General Instructions

The U.S. Special Forces Physical Conditioning Program runs five consecutive days per week for twelve consecutive weeks. Once you begin the program, *you should maintain the built-in momentum of the program.* That is, you should resist any excuse (be it fatigue, sore muscles, self-pity, or bad weather) for any kind of lapse, no matter how brief you convince yourself that lapse will be.

During the early stages of this program, you may find yourself feeling "down" or slightly depressed. This is normal, because you will be making demands on a body that may be somewhat reluctant to be demanded upon; and reluctant bodies, you will soon discover (if you haven't already), have a whole bagful of tricks at their disposal to get you to cease your demands upon them—one of which is to give you a good case of the blahs. However, if you stick *strictly* to the schedules, any blahs will eventually give way to feelings of vitality and confidence. In other words, the discomfort you feel in the early stages of this program may be psychological as well as physical. Be prepared to combat both. One important thing you should do in this regard is to get plenty of rest; make it a habit to get two hours of sleep before midnight (in order to keep your sleep clock synchronized with your biological clock).

Between one and two hours will be required per day to complete the quotas for both the calisthenics and the running. The time required progresses with the demands of the program.

Choose a training time that is best for you, considering your personal circumstances, but be sure it is one you can depend on having available to you on a *regular* basis. Certainly the best time of day for the kind of training called for in this program is the morning, especially the early morning, before the demands of the day have taken their toll in energy and resolve; but any time of day is fine as long as it is available to you on a regular basis.

Stretching

Before beginning each session of calisthenics and running, you should gently stretch out the muscles you will be exercising. This book includes a comprehensive stretching program, based on the famous Penn State Flexibility Program, for just this purpose. The Stretching Program consists of fourteen individual stretching exercises.

Comprehensive stretching provides three major benefits: (1) it helps prevent injury (muscle tears); (2) it aids the overall conditioning process; and (3) it enhances athletic flexibility.

To take maximum advantage of these stretching benefits, you should begin the scheduled calisthenics session as soon after you finish the stretching exercises as possible; and then follow the calisthenics session almost immediately with the scheduled conditioning hike (the run/sprint/walk)—that is, while your muscles are still fully stretched. If your circumstances do not permit an immediate succession from the calisthenics session to the conditioning hike, then be sure to do a minimum of two minutes of additional stretching before you run, concentrating on the exercises (such as the Toe Touch, the Trailer, the Hurdler's Stretch, and the Ninety-Degree Groin Stretch) that stretch the leg and groin muscles.

In addition to stretching out before each workout, you should also stretch out after each workout. Comprehensive after-workout stretching can help prevent, or at least lessen the severity of, soreness and stiffness in the muscles.

See Table 1 for complete schedules for both before-work-out and after-workout stretching.

Diet

Your body will need a complete, consistent, and *balanced* supply of nutrients in order to function properly, as well as build itself up, during the training process; it will also need plenty of liquids—*water* being the best of all. Here are some specific recommendations:

- Pick up a good book on nutrition at the local library or bookstore and read it. (Keep it in the john and read a little of it each day.) And put this little truism on your bathroom mirror: A balanced, intelligent diet is as important to the true athlete as a balanced, intelligent conditioning program. (The book I keep in my john is *Jane Brody's Nutrition Book*.)
- Many people believe they have to eat a lot of red meat (beef, especially) in order to be athletic. They associate red meat (and more generally, protein) with muscle development. The truth is, however, that if you do eat a lot of meat—that is, more than your body needs—about the only thing you're going to develop is your waistline. There are two reasons for this: (1) meat from domesticated animals today tends to contain a high proportion of fat; and (2) the body converts to fat any protein it does not have immediate need for. Many serious athletes eat very little red meat at all, seeking protein instead in such low-fat sources as fish, poultry, legumes (beans and peas), grains, and natural yogurt. Nuts are another good source of protein; in fact, you may wish to keep a jar of unsalted, dry-roasted pea-nuts around for snacking.
- Consider taking a vitamin-and-mineral supplement on a regular basis. I used to pooh-pooh doing that sort of thing (back in my invincible days), then I started

taking them. The differences I began to notice—including greater stamina, and fewer and shorter incidences of colds and the flu—may have been largely coincidental, or psychological, but I don't think so. If you're a junk-food addict, or if you take no more than "thank you, ma'am" helpings of vegetables and fruit, there is no question that you should take a vitamin-and-mineral supplement. (*Caution:* I do *not* recommend vitamin megadosing, or any other form of "if one is good, a hundred is better" mentality.) Here's a mail-order source for high-quality, relatively low-cost vitamin and mineral supplements: Puritan's Pride, 105 Orville Drive, Bohemia, NY 11716 (ask for their catalog).

- Avoid dosing yourself with sugar just before an exercise session; in other words, no candy bars or soft drinks. Abrupt injections of sugar into your system will tend to do more harm than good. For energy, rely on the carbohydrates contained in such foods as whole wheat bread, pasta, and potatoes. In fact, avoid heavily sugared foods altogether (yes, including ice cream).
- Avoid taking alcoholic beverages immediately before or after a workout session. Reacquaint yourself with water—and drink *plenty* of it.
- If you intend to diet in conjunction with engaging in this conditioning program, do not go on any kind of severe or "crash" diet. Instead, concentrate on isolating bad eating habits and trying to break them (keeping in mind it takes approximately twenty-one days to break an old habit).
- On the other hand, avoid using this conditioning program as an excuse to start drinking an extra beer or two, or eating those chocolate-drenched doughnuts you've conscientiously been denying yourself—up until now.
- If you're looking around for a mate, consider marrying a nutritionist.

Sore Muscles

You will undoubtedly experience at least some soreness and stiffness in *several* of your body's major and minor muscles during the first days, perhaps even weeks, of fulfilling the requirements of this program. This is a normal occurrence. Just how much soreness and stiffness you experience will depend largely on the condition of your muscles at the time you begin the program, and how much stretching you do before and after each workout.

Unfortunately, it is also a normal occurrence to use sore muscles as an excuse to "take the day off." You should avoid this for two very good reasons. One, it's too easy to lose your momentum: a one-day lapse becomes a two-day lapse that becomes—you know the story, I'm sure. And two, for this program to be fully effective, you must keep pressuring your muscles to become stronger and more enduring. And you must keep signaling them that their tactic of making you uncomfortable as a way of getting you to stop taxing them isn't going to work. In fact, the quickest way to get rid of soreness or stiffness in any muscle is to use that muscle. In other words, the best tactic to use on a complaining muscle is the same one that works best on a complaining child: give it some work to do.

You can sometimes avoid getting soreness and stiffness in your muscles, or at least keep the degree of discomfort down, by keeping yourself warm and as active and mobile as possible after each workout. Perhaps the single most beneficial thing you can do is at least two to three minutes of stretching after each workout. For a formal program of after-workout stretching, refer to the Stretching Program in this book.

To soothe sore muscles, draw a warm bath and indulge yourself.

Shoes/Foot Care

To maximize the effectiveness of the Running Program, as well as that of several of the individual calisthenic exercises, it is *strongly* recommended that you wear heavy boots (combat or jump boots, or the like). The heavy boots provide additional weight that must be compensated for with additional effort on your part. This additional weight pressures your leg muscles to become stronger and more enduring at a faster rate. Combat boots and jump boots are available at most Army surplus stores. As an alternative, you may wish to try wearing ankle weights.

If heavy boots are not in the picture for you, use well-fitting running shoes for the Running Program. And do not skimp on them; spend what you need to spend for good quality and for proper fit and support. If you tend to pronate, get shoes that provide protection against pronation. If you're not sure exactly what kind of support you need, you may wish to obtain shoes that offer more support than you may actually need—that is, to be safe rather than sorry. (Ask the sales clerk for a recommendation, explaining what you intend to use your shoes for. But *first,* ask the clerk if he or she is a runner.) I use New Balance 565's for training, and Nike Pegasus for running marathons and road races; but I am not a pronator.

If you opt for the heavy boots, you may wish to wear two pairs of cotton athletic socks (or fit half-inch foam-rubber pads inside the boots) to help prevent blisters. Even then, it is not always possible to prevent friction blisters, especially if your boots are new and stiff. If you do develop a blister at any point, place an ice-cold compress on the affected area just as soon as possible. Then, to prevent further irritation, place a doughnut-shaped moleskin wafer around, *but not on,* the affected area (you can purchase moleskin at any drug store), or wrap the affected area in half-inch foam rubber.

Getting Started

As a starting point, read through the Calisthenics Program
and attempt a few repetitions of each exercise as you go.
Earmark the more difficult exercises, then return to those for
additional practice—and try not to be discouraged if you find
you have a book full of earmarks! Learn all the exercises, at
least the proper positionings of the individual steps, before
you formally engage in the daily schedules. Note from Table
2, however, that you are not scheduled to execute some of
the exercises until you are already into the program. There is
no reason to worry, therefore, if you find you are unable to
perform any of the more difficult exercises prior to formally
beginning the program. In fact, the exercises you can perform will help prepare your muscles for executing the more
difficult exercises later on.

There is, by the way, a definite difference between learning
the exercises and mastering them. Learn how to do the
exercises before you formally begin the program; then attempt to master the exercises as you progress through the
program.

For further starting tips, refer to Week 0 in the Schedules
section on page 137.

Keeping Count

It is important to maintain an audible step-and-cycle count
during each scheduled exercise. Maintaining an audible count
will help you sustain the proper rhythm and help you keep
track of the number of cycles performed; it will also, you will
soon discover, place an additional burden on you—provided
you keep count at a forceful decibel level—to be overcome
with additional effort (to your benefit). The following example demonstrates how you should keep count.

If the exercise being performed is a four-step exercise, you count the first cycle as follows: ONE, TWO, THREE, *ONE*. You then count the second cycle: ONE, TWO, THREE, *TWO*. The third: ONE, TWO, THREE, *THREE*. And so on, up to the tenth cycle. At the eleventh cycle, you restart the cycle count at ONE, and then count up to TWENTY; at the twenty-first cycle, you restart the cycle count at ONE again, and then count up to THIRTY; and so forth.

You will find yourself tempted, especially during moments of high stress, to keep count either in a whisper or with no audible utterance at all. To get maximum benefit from each exercise, resist this temptation as best you can. Count as if to cause the world to stand up and take notice of you.

Keeping at It

Among life's hard little truths is that erratic or halfhearted physical conditioning is nearly as worthless as no conditioning at all. Therefore, commit yourself from the very beginning of this program to exacting standards of performance (to doing the Push-Up *correctly,* for example) and to regular and inflexible training habits: neither rain nor sleet nor sore, aching, reluctant muscles should stay you from your appointed daily schedule of sweat and strain. You will find the rewards well worth your exacting standards.

Preventing Injuries

There are two very important things you can do to help prevent injuries during the course of this, or any other, physical conditioning: (1) stretch out properly before each workout, and (2) know as much about the causes of injury, and about your body in relation to these causes, as possible.

To stretch out properly, you should use *religiously* the Stretching Program presented in the next section of this book. To learn about the causes of injury, add to your list of books recently read a sports physiology book such as Ken Sprague's *The Athlete's Body* (this book is nontechnical and reads quickly).

Believe me: the *last* thing you want is to get seven or eight weeks into this program and find yourself on the injured reserve list—out for the season. So take care of yourself—by being smart.

The Stretching Program

This section provides a comprehensive stretching program, and includes separate schedules for *before*-workout stretching and *after*-workout stretching. These schedules require only a little over five minutes and two minutes respectively to complete (see Table 1 on page 30).

Comprehensive before-workout stretching serves three major purposes:

- It helps prevent injury (muscle tears).
- It aids the overall conditioning process.
- It enhances athletic flexibility.

Comprehensive after-workout stretching helps prevent muscles from becoming sore and stiff.

There are fourteen individual exercises in the Stretching Program. Each step of any one exercise requires only ten seconds to complete.

Note • The Stretching Program is not a part of the Navy conditioning program on which the rest of this book is based. It was developed by the author in consultation with the attending physician for the University of New Hampshire football and basketball teams. Essentially, it is an enhancement of the flexibility program used by the Penn State football team.

In performing the following exercises, *do not* apply pressure to your muscles to the point of feeling pain; pain is injury. Apply pressure only to the point where you can feel a mild tension in your muscles, and increase the pressure only as you are able to without incurring pain.

1. Neck Stretch

Muscles Stretched • Neck muscles.

Starting Position • Standing at the position of attention, place the feet comfortably apart, about three to four inches. Place the palms of the hands against the back of the head, fingers interlaced, elbows pressed backward.

Execution • PULL IT FORWARD   Pull the head forward, placing a mild stretch on the muscles in the back of the neck. Hold for ten seconds.

PUSH IT BACK   Move the palms to the forehead, fingers interlaced, and push the head backward, placing a mild stretch on the muscles in the front of the neck. Hold for ten seconds.

PULL IT LEFT   Straightening the head, grasp the right side of the head with the left hand. Pull the head to the left, placing a mild stretch on the muscles in the right side of the neck. Hold for ten seconds.

PULL IT RIGHT   Straightening the head, grasp the left side of the head with the right hand. Pull the head to the right, placing a mild stretch on the muscles in the left side of the neck. Hold for ten seconds.

LOOK LEFT   Straightening the head, turn the head to the left as far as possible. Hold for ten seconds.

LOOK RIGHT   Turn the head to the right as far as possible. Hold for ten seconds.

Comments • The total time for this one is only sixty seconds. Keep time by counting the seconds as thousands: "One thousand. Two thousand. Three thousand . . ."

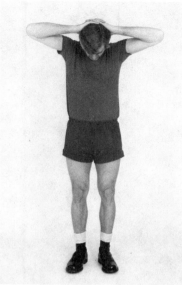
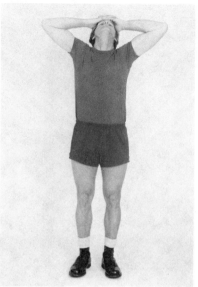

(Neck Stretch) Pull it forward   Push it back

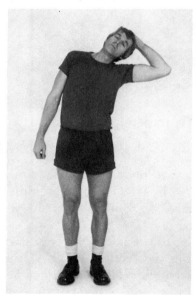
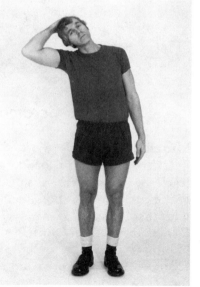

Pull it left   Pull it right

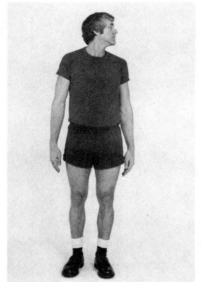
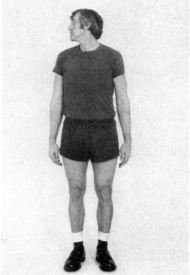

Look left   Look right

2. Scratch Your Back

Muscles Stretched • Side.

Starting Position • Standing at the position of attention, reach the extended fingers of the right hand down the middle of the back as far as possible. Grasp the doubled right elbow with the left hand.

Execution • LEAN LEFT Lean to the left as far as possible, placing a mild stretch on the right side. Hold for ten seconds; then straighten and reverse the relative positions of the arms: reach the left extended fingers down the back and grasp the left elbow with the right hand.

LEAN RIGHT Lean to the right as far as possible, placing a mild stretch on the left side. Hold for ten seconds.

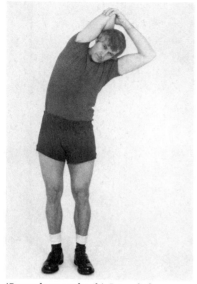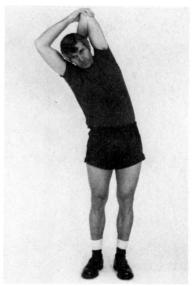

(Scratch your back) Lean left   Lean right

3. Handcuff

Muscles Stretched • Shoulder girdle.
Starting Position • Standing at the position of attention, place the arms behind the back and interlock the fingers, palm to palm. Extend the arms.
Execution • LIFT Slowly lift the arms until you feel a mild stretch in the shoulders. Hold for ten seconds.

4. Toe Touch

Muscles Stretched • Hamstrings.
Starting Position • Standing at the position of attention, place the feet comfortably apart, about three to four inches. Lock the knees, then bend forward at the waist until the trunk is approximately parallel to the ground. Relax, with the arms dangling.
Execution • TOUCH YOUR TOES Slowly reach the fingertips toward the toes, placing a mild stretch behind the

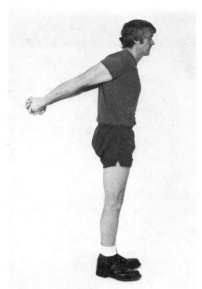

(Handcuff) Lift

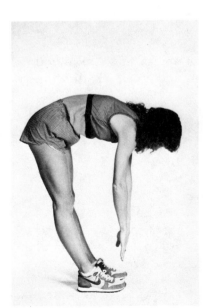

(Toe Touch) Starting position

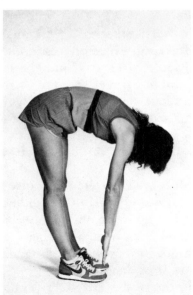

Touch your toes. Do it again

knees. Actually touch the toes only if you are able to with relative ease (no pain behind the knees). Hold for ten seconds; then relax (still bending forward).

DO IT AGAIN Repeating the previous step, attempt to reach farther toward the ground. The ultimate goal of this step is to place the palms of the hands flat on the ground. Hold for ten seconds.

Comments • Reach and stretch smoothly; that is, do not bounce.

Work up gradually to the goals (touching the toes; placing the palms flat on the ground).

5. Trailer

Muscles Stretched • Hamstrings.
Starting Position • In a standing position, step over the left foot with the right foot, crossing the legs at the knees, and place the right foot at the left side of the left foot. Align the toes of both feet.
Execution • TOUCH YOUR RIGHT TOES Bending at the waist, reach toward the toes of the right foot, placing a mild stretch on the hamstrings. Hold for ten seconds. Then reverse the relative positions of the feet and legs: place the left foot at the right side of the right foot, aligning the toes.

TOUCH YOUR LEFT TOES Bending at the waist, reach toward the toes of the left foot, placing a mild stretch on the hamstrings. Hold for ten seconds.

6. Grab It

Muscles Stretched • Lower and upper back, hamstrings, calves.
Starting Position • In a sitting position, spread the legs about eighteen inches apart. Point the toes up.
Execution • GRAB YOUR ANKLES Reach toward the

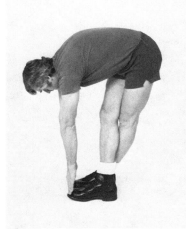
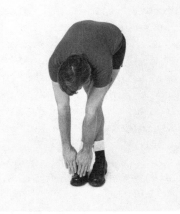

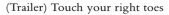

(Trailer) Touch your right toes   Touch your left toes

ankles, grasping them *only* if you are able to without pain.
Hold for ten seconds, then release them.

GRAB YOUR TOES Reach toward the toes, grasping
them *only* if you are able to without pain. Hold for ten
seconds, then release them.

GRAB YOUR INSTEPS Reach toward the insteps,
again grasping them only if you are able to without pain.
Hold for about ten seconds.

Comments • Keep the toes pointed up, the knees locked.

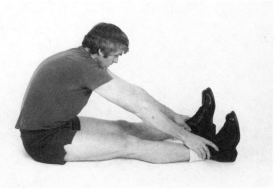

(Grab It) Grab your ankles

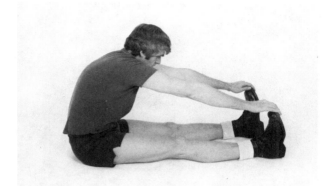

Grab your toes

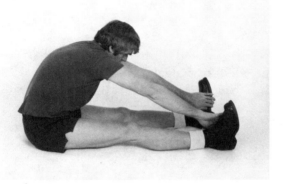

Grab your insteps

7. Butterfly

Muscles Stretched • Groin, lower back, upper back.

Starting Position • In a sitting position, bend the knees outward until the soles of the feet are flush together. Pull the touching feet as far toward the groin as possible. Grasp the ends of the feet.

Execution • PULL Pulling the trunk forward with the arms, press the forehead toward the feet. Simultaneously press the knees toward the ground. When you feel a mild stretch in the groin, hold for ten seconds.

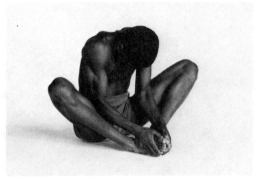

(Butterfly) Pull

Comments • The goal with this one is to be able to hold the forehead all the way down against the feet while holding the legs flat on the ground. Strive toward this goal gradually. And gently.

8. Spinal Twist

Muscles Stretched • Lower and upper back, hips.
Starting Position • In a sitting position, rest backward on the extended arms and extend the legs directly forward. Bending the right knee, cross the right leg over the left leg and place the right foot flat on the ground. The right ankle is now resting against the left thigh, just above the knee. Twisting the trunk to the right, rest the left elbow against the right thigh, just above the knee.
Execution • TWIST RIGHT   Pushing against the right leg with the left elbow, twist the trunk to the right. When you can feel a mild stretch in the lower and upper back muscles, hold for ten seconds. Release, then reverse the relative positions of the arms and legs: leaning backward on the left arm, cross the left leg over the extended right leg; rest the right elbow against the left thigh, just above the knee.

TWIST LEFT   Pushing against the left leg with the right arm, twist the trunk to the left. When you can feel a mild stretch on the lower and upper back muscles, hold for ten seconds.

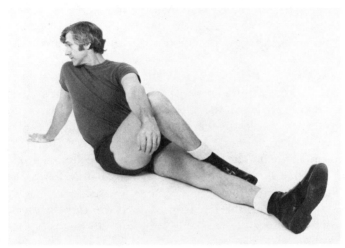

(Spinal Twist) Twist right

Twist left

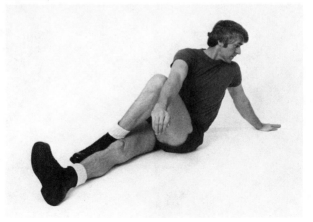

9. Foot to Axilla

Muscles Stretched • Hips.

Starting Position • In a sitting position, extend the legs directly forward. Bending and elevating the right leg, grasp the foot with the left hand and the upper ankle with the right hand. Press the cradle of the bent right elbow against the elevated knee.

Execution • RIGHT FOOT   Pull the right foot toward the left armpit, and simultaneously pull (with the arm and elbow) the knee toward the chest. When you feel a mild stretch in the hips, hold for ten seconds. Release, then reverse the relative positions of the legs and arms: extend the right leg; bend and elevate the left leg, grasping the upper ankle with the left hand, the foot with the right hand. Press the cradle of the left bent elbow against the elevated knee.

LEFT FOOT   Pull the left foot toward the right armpit, and simultaneously pull (with the arm and elbow) the knee toward the chest. When you feel a mild stretch in the hips, hold for ten seconds.

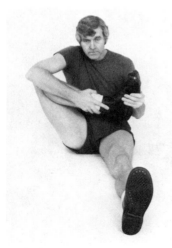
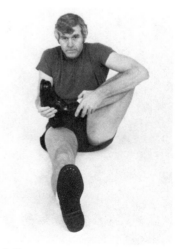

Right foot   Left foot

10. Sole to Thigh

Muscles Stretched • Back, hamstrings, groin.
Starting Position • In a sitting position, extend the legs directly forward. Bending the right knee, pull the right sole along the inside of the left leg as far toward the groin as possible; then bend forward at the waist and grasp the left ankle with both hands. Keep the toes of the left foot pointed upward.
Execution • RIGHT SOLE   Pull the trunk forward, placing a mild stretch on the back and hamstrings. Hold for ten seconds; then release and reverse the relative positions of the arms and legs: extend the right leg; reach forward and grasp the right ankle with both hands, simultaneously bending the left knee and sliding the sole along the inside of the right leg as far toward the groin as possible.

   LEFT SOLE   Pull the trunk forward, placing a mild stretch on the back and hamstrings. Hold for ten seconds.

11. Legs Over

Muscles Stretched • Lower back, hamstrings.
Starting Position • Lying on the ground, legs spread about eighteen inches apart, rotate the legs over the trunk and head so that you are lying on the shoulders and upper back. Grasp the toes with the hands, and straighten the legs.
Execution • PULL YOUR TOES   Pull the toes toward the ground, placing a mild stretch on the lower back and hamstrings. Keep the legs as straight as possible. Hold for ten seconds.
Comments • If necessary, begin the exercise with the legs slightly bent; then gradually straighten the legs, while pulling the toes toward the ground.

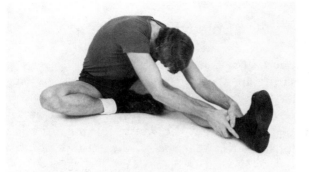

(Sole to Thigh) Right sole

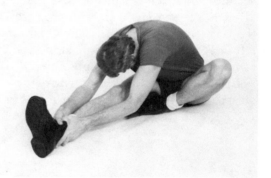

Left sole

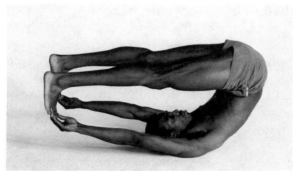

(Legs Over) Pull your toes

12. Sit Up and Reach Out

Muscles Stretched • Lower and upper back.
Starting Position • In a sitting position, spread the legs as far apart as possible. Point the toes outward.
Execution • DOWN THE MIDDLE Bending at the waist, reach forward and rest the palms of the hands on the ground, placing a mild stretch on the back and the legs. Hold for ten seconds; then release. Straighten the back.

REACH RIGHT Reaching down the right leg, attempt to touch the nose to the right knee. When you feel a mild stretch, hold for ten seconds. Release; straighten the back.

REACH LEFT Reaching down the left leg, attempt to touch the nose to the left knee. When you feel a mild stretch, hold for ten seconds.

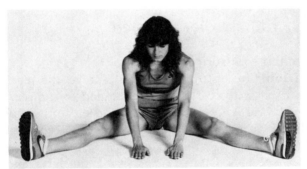

Down the middle

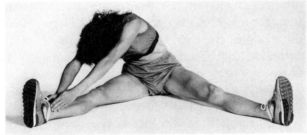

Reach right

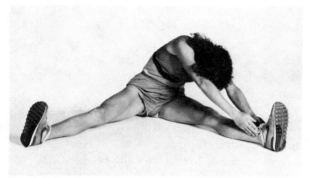

Reach left

13. Hurdler's Stretch

Muscles Stretched • Quadriceps.

Starting Position • In a sitting position, spread the legs. Supporting yourself with the left arm extended to the rear, and pulling on the right foot, bend the right leg until fully doubled, with the toes pointing directly to the rear, heel against buttock.

Execution • LEAN ON RIGHT Allowing the left hand to slide backward, gradually lean backward, placing an increasing stretch on the quadriceps, until the back is touching the ground. Hold for ten seconds. Then reverse the relative positions of the legs: supporting yourself with the right arm extended to the rear, bend the left leg until fully doubled, with the toes pointing directly to the rear, heel against buttock.

LEAN ON LEFT Allowing the right hand to slide backward, gradually lean backward, placing an increasing stretch on the quadriceps, until the back is touching the ground. Hold for ten seconds.

Comments • At first, you may not be able to ease the back all the way to the ground. If you aren't, be patient—don't push it; stop at the point your knee begins to rise from the ground. Simply attempt to stretch a little farther each time you perform the exercise.

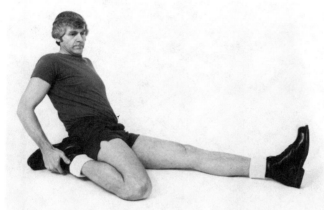

(Hurdler's Stretch) Starting position

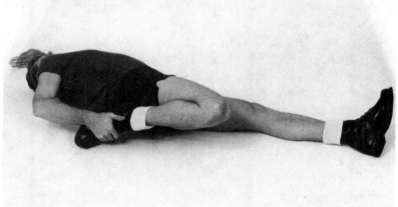

Lean on right

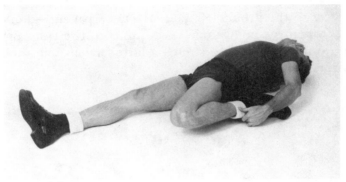

Lean on left

14. Ninety-Degree Groin Stretch

Muscles Stretched • Groin.

Starting Position • From the position of attention, turn the right foot clockwise until at a ninety-degree angle with the left foot. Stepping rightward, position the right foot three to four feet from the left foot. Face in the same direction in which the right foot is pointing.

Execution • LEAN RIGHT   Bending the right knee, lean in the plane of the right leg, placing a mild stretch on the groin. Hold for ten seconds. Then reverse the relative position of the legs: place the left foot at a ninety-degree angle with the right foot and step leftward three to four feet.

LEAN LEFT   Bending the left knee, lean in the plane of the left leg, placing a mild stretch on the groin. Hold for ten seconds.

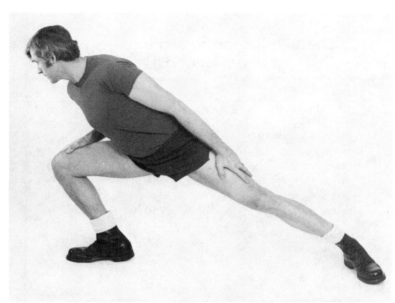

(Ninety-Degree Groin Stretch) Lean right

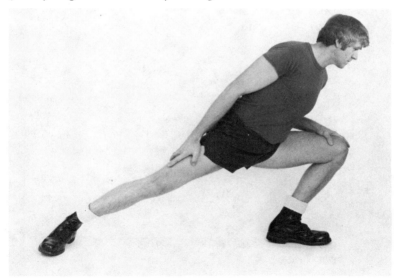

Lean left

Table 1:
Schedule for the Stretching Program
(in seconds)

Exercise	Before-Workout	After-Workout
1. Neck Stretch		
PULL IT FORWARD	10	0
PUSH IT BACK	10	0
PULL IT LEFT	10	0
PULL IT RIGHT	10	0
LOOK LEFT	10	0
LOOK RIGHT	10	0
2. Scratch Your Back		
LEAN LEFT	10	5
LEAN RIGHT	10	5
3. Handcuff		
LIFT	10	5
4. Toe Touch		
TOUCH YOUR TOES	10	5
DO IT AGAIN	10	5
5. Trailer		
TOUCH YOUR RIGHT TOES	10	5
TOUCH YOUR LEFT TOES	10	5
6. Grab It		
GRAB YOUR ANKLES	10	5
GRAB YOUR TOES	10	5
GRAB YOUR INSTEPS	10	5
7. Butterfly		
PULL	10	5
8. Spinal Twist		
TWIST RIGHT	10	5
TWIST LEFT	10	5

Table 1 (cont'd)

Exercise	Before-Workout	After-Workout
9. Foot to Axilla		
RIGHT FOOT	10	5
LEFT FOOT	10	5
10. Sole to Thigh		
RIGHT SOLE	10	5
LEFT SOLE	10	5
11. Legs Over		
PULL YOUR TOES	10	5
12. Sit Up and Reach Out		
DOWN THE MIDDLE	10	5
REACH RIGHT	10	5
REACH LEFT	10	5
13. Hurdler's Stretch		
LEAN ON RIGHT	10	5
LEAN ON LEFT	10	5
14. Ninety-Degree Groin Stretch		
LEAN RIGHT	10	5
LEAN LEFT	10	5
Total Time	5 min. 10 sec.	2 min. 5 sec.

The Calisthenics Program

The Calisthenics Program is designed to enhance the strength, agility, and endurance of nearly every "action" muscle in the human body. The program consists of a comprehensive group of forty-six individual exercises, targeted toward five general body areas, and a twelve-week schedule of daily exercising. The forty-six exercises are presented and discussed in detail in the following pages, and are grouped under five categories: (1) The General Warm-Up Exercises (involving all body areas); (2) The Abdominal Exercises; (3) The Side and Oblique Exercises; (4) The Leg and Groin Exercises; and (5) The Arm, Chest, and Shoulder Exercises.

With *comprehensive* and *redundant* body coverage, these forty-six exercises will strengthen every muscle you will ever need to use in a competitive situation; but perhaps even more importantly, they will enhance your ability to use your strength in complex and coordinated ways—that is, with the agility of the true athlete. In addition, these exercises will tone your muscles to give you that distinctive "athletic" look.

A twelve-week schedule for the Calisthenics Program is provided at the end of this section (Table 2, page 126). Week-by-week schedules are provided in the section entitled Schedules.

Procedures and Techniques

For psychological as well as practical considerations, it is recommended that you undertake the Calisthenics Program with at least one other person. Not only does misery like company, not to mention find it distracting, but four of the exercises are best performed in two-person teams. (These four exercises can be performed without assistance, however, if necessary.) Having a partner will also help you adhere strictly to the training schedule.

Learn one exercise at a time, step by step, concentrating your efforts on the more difficult exercises. Some of the exercises—in particular, the Stomach Stretcher, the Groin Stretcher, and the Flutter Kick—may take a little time to get the hang of. Work persistently at these until you conquer them. Even many frogman and SEAL trainees have difficulty mastering these more difficult exercises, so don't get discouraged. Begin the Calisthenics Program only after you are able to perform at least the first quota listed for each exercise included in Session 1 (see Table 2, or see Week 1 under Schedules). Several of the exercises are not scheduled to be performed formally until later in the program (for example, the Leg Lever, the Sitting Knee Bend, and the One-Legged Sit-Up). Try all of these exercises, too; but do not be concerned about being able to perform them properly until you have progressed to them in the schedule.

If you would honestly rate your current state of physical condition as "pretty bad," you may wish to engage in two weeks of preconditioning before undertaking the formal program. If you choose to do this, on each day of the first week (five days), do half the quotas listed under Session 1; on each day of the second week, do half the quotas listed under Session 2. In addition, run for six consecutive minutes (that is, without walking) each day of the first week, and for eight consecutive minutes each day of the second week. Then begin the formal program, starting with the full exercise and running quotas listed for Session 1.

You should execute the exercises scheduled for any one session in the order in which they are listed, and in rapid succession; that is, with no more than a one-minute pause between any two exercises. During any pause, high-step (run, bringing your knees up as high as possible) either in place or around the circumference of any circle that brings you back to your starting point. In other words, keep moving at all times, to keep a relentless demand on both lung and limb. (The whole secret to this program is to do it *right*, and give it your all.)

Some of the exercises in the Calisthenics Program (such as the Regulation Sit-Up) require you to exercise on your back. To prevent any chafing to the lower back (tailbone) area when performing these exercises, you may wish to lie on some kind of padding (folded blanket, floor mat). This is especially true for those of you, like me, who have no "buns."

For added inspiration, you may wish to play some rousing music while you are performing the calisthenic exercises. If you have a portable cassette player/recorder, make some tapes of whatever raises gooseflesh up and down your arms. And play it *loud*.

The General Warm-Up Exercises

1. Full Jumping Jack
2. Half Jumping Jack
3. Side Twister Stretcher
4. Trunk Rotation
5. Trunk Bending Fore and Aft
6. Trunk Twister
7. Windmill, Four-count
8. Windmill, Two-count
9. Trunk Side Stretcher
10. Rocking Chair

The General Warm-Up Exercises are designed to stimulate the circulatory and respiratory systems; to generally stretch out the muscles, especially those that may be sore and stiff from previous workout sessions; and to ease into the proper mental attitude necessary for rigorous and demanding use of the body systems. In effect, they "get you into the groove."

The General Warm-Up Exercises also participate significantly in the process of strengthening the muscles and enhancing overall agility. They do this by causing you to move body mass through space (or resist the force of gravity), often in ways that require coordination, flexibility, and balance.

1. Full Jumping Jack

Starting Position • Stand fully erect (at the position of attention) with the elbows locked at the sides; extend the fingers downward. Keep the head up, eyes forward.

Execution • ONE While jumping, spread the legs apart so that the feet strike the ground about twelve to eighteen inches from their respective starting positions; simultaneously rotate the arms upward until the thumbs of each hand touch over the head. The feet are now spread from two to three feet apart; the arms are *fully* extended over the head; the fingers are still fully extended.

TWO Recover to the starting position by reversing the ONE count: while jumping, bring the legs together, simultaneously rotating the locked arms back to the sides (without slapping the sides). You are now ready for the ONE count of the next cycle.

Comments • Breathe deeply, but not forcibly, throughout the exercise. Forced breathing (hyperventilation), as well as holding the breath (hypoventilation), may bring on dizziness and untimely fatigue. Breathe in sympathy with what your body requires at the moment.

Don't forget to count audibly on the execution of each step: "ONE, *ONE—ONE, TWO—ONE, THREE* . . .

ONE, *TEN*—ONE, *ONE*—ONE, *TWO* . . . ONE,
TWENTY . . . ," and so on.

Jump off, and land on, the balls of your feet. Avoid
bending the elbows at any time. Maintain a rapid pace.

The Full Jumping Jack serves primarily to get the heart and
lungs out of first gear and into second. However, as do all the
other exercises in the Calisthenics Program, the Full Jumping
Jack also participates in strengthening the muscles it involves
(leg and arm muscles, in this case), by placing a load on
them—that is, by forcing them to move body mass through
space.

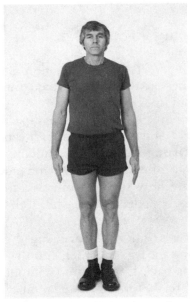
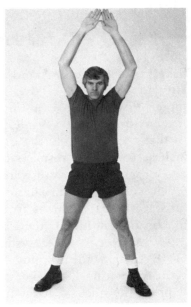

(Full Jumping Jack) Starting and   One
recovery position

2. Half Jumping Jack

Starting Position • Same as for Full Jumping Jack: stand at
the position of attention with the elbows locked at the sides,
fingers extended; keep the head up, eyes forward.

Execution • ONE   Jumping upward, spread the legs apart

so that the feet strike the ground about nine to twelve inches from their respective starting positions; simultaneously rotate the arms upward until they are straight out from the sides (parallel to the ground). The feet are now about one-half to two-thirds as far apart as they are at the end of the ONE count of the Full Jumping Jack; the arms and fingers are fully extended, parallel to the ground. The head is up; the eyes are forward.

TWO Recover to the starting position by reversing the ONE count: jumping upward, bring the legs together while simultaneously lowering the arms smoothly back to the sides (without slapping the sides). You are now ready for the ONE count of the next cycle.

Comments • Begin the Half Jumping Jack at a moderate pace, then increase the tempo until you are executing as rapidly as possible. Toward the end, you should be a blur of activity to an outside observer.

You may find yourself holding your breath during this exercise. Try not to. And remember to count audibly on the execution of each step.

Jump off, and land on, the balls of your feet. Keep your arms fully extended (they may have a tendency to sag, especially as the tempo increases).

Whereas the Full Jumping Jack puts the heart and lungs into second gear, the Half Jumping Jack puts them into third (or fourth!).

3. Side Twister Stretcher

Starting Position • Place the right wrist over the left wrist and twist the wrists inward until the hands are palm to palm; interlock the fingers. Extend the arms as far over the head as possible and squeeze the upper arms against the sides of the head. This contortion may be a little uncomfortable at first, but bear with it; the muscles in the arms and shoulders will eventually stretch and adjust. Stand with the trunk erect and the feet spread three to four feet apart. Firmly lock the knees.

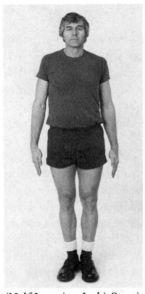 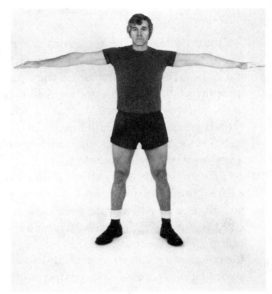

(Half Jumping Jack) Starting
and recovery position

One

Execution • ONE   Twist the trunk smoothly leftward, until you are facing in the direction in which the left foot is pointing, then bend down vigorously from the waist until the interlocked fingers touch the left toes. Keep the fingers firmly interlocked and the arms extended—and *keep the knees firmly locked*. If at first you are unable to touch the toes, reach toward them, but without bouncing.

TWO   Recover to the starting position by smoothly lifting the trunk upward and then twisting it to face forward.

THREE   Twist the trunk smoothly rightward, until you are facing in the direction in which the right foot is pointing, then bend down vigorously from the waist until the interlocked fingers touch the right toes. Keep the knees firmly locked. If unable to touch the toes, reach toward them, again without bouncing.

FOUR   Recover to the starting position by smoothly lifting the trunk upward and then twisting it to face forward.

Comments • Concentrate on form and technique. Resist any tendency to bend the knees on the ONE and THREE counts, and keep the fingers snugly interlocked and the arms as fully extended as possible. Keeping firm pressure against the sides of your head with your arms will help you maintain proper form.

At first, you will probably experience intense pressure in the knee region on the ONE and THREE counts. If you keep reaching toward the toes, eventually your muscles will stretch out and this pressure will lessen.

Remember to count audibly on the execution of each step, and to breathe naturally.

The Side Twister Stretcher is primarily a stretching exercise; however, unlike the stretching exercises in the Stretching Program, which are static exercises, the Side Twister Stretcher is a dynamic exercise—that is, it involves movement of body mass through space, while requiring you to maintain balance, form, and rhythm. Therefore, not only does the Side Twister Stretcher serve to stretch out muscles (in the sides, legs, and arms); it also serves to strengthen muscles, *and* to enhance your coordination and balance skills—and thus overall agility.

This is true of all the other exercises in this grouping.

4. Trunk Rotation

Starting Position • Stand at the position of attention with the hands on the hips, fingers forward, thumbs rearward. Lock the knees.

Execution • ONE   Bend the trunk forward at the waist until the head is as close to the ground as you can get it. You should feel fairly intense pressure behind the knee area. Keep the knees firmly locked and the legs rigidly straight.

TWO   Rotate the trunk smoothly rightward and lean as far directly to the right as you can. You should feel pressure in the pelvic and lower back areas.

THREE   Rotate the trunk smoothly rearward and lean as far directly to the rear as you can. You should feel pressure in the lower back and stomach areas. (To get an idea of what

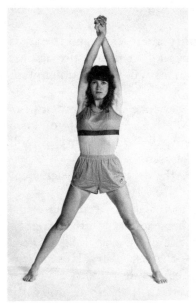

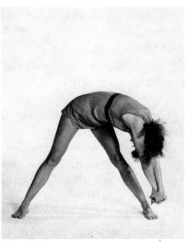

(Side Twister Stretcher) Starting and recovery position

One

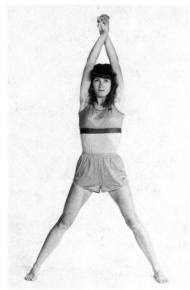

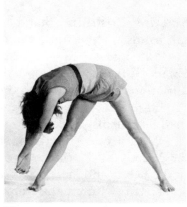

Two

Three

this exercise is doing, press your stomach area with a finger at this point.)

FOUR   Rotate the trunk smoothly leftward and lean as far directly to the left as you can.

Comments • On the ONE count of the second cycle (and on the ONE count of every cycle thereafter), rotate the trunk forward and lean as far directly forward as you can.

Execute at a moderate rate during the first week or so; then gradually increase the tempo, but without losing control of form and technique. Be sure to keep your knees locked and legs straight throughout the exercise.

Halfway through the daily quota, reverse the direction of motion; that is, move the trunk to the left on the ONE count instead of to the right.

As with the Side Twister Stretcher, you are stretching muscles here, but you are also strengthening muscles, and enhancing agility.

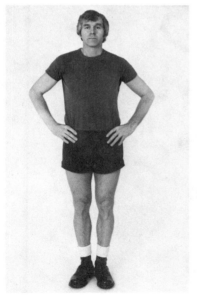

(Trunk Rotation) Starting position

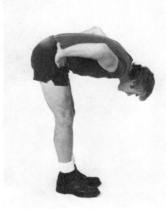

One

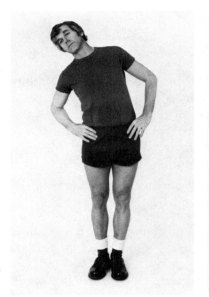

Two

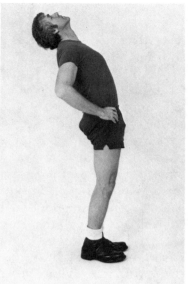

Three

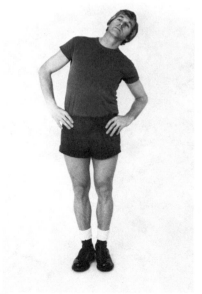

Four

5. Trunk Bending Fore and Aft

Starting Position • Stand at the position of attention with the hands on the hips, fingers forward, thumbs rearward. Lock the knees.

Execution • ONE Bend the trunk smoothly forward at the waist and as far toward the ground as possible. As with the Trunk Rotation, you should feel fairly intense pressure behind the knee area. Keep the knees firmly locked and the legs straight.

TWO Recover to the starting position by lifting the trunk smoothly upward.

THREE Bend the trunk directly backward and lean as far to the rear as possible. (Feel the thigh and stomach muscles at this point.)

FOUR Recover to the starting position by bending the trunk smoothly forward.

Comments • Bend as far forward and as far rearward as you can, but keep the knees locked and the feet firmly planted on the ground.

Trunk Bending is another good stretcher and simultaneous strengthener. Note that there is a great deal of built-in redundancy among these exercises—once is never enough!

6. Trunk Twister

Starting Position • Standing at the position of attention, place the feet a comfortable distance apart—about six to eight inches. Place the upper part of the fingers against the back of the head, palms facing inward, so that the middle fingers just touch. (The fingers are parallel to the ground.) Keep the elbows pressed rearward.

Execution • ONE Twist the trunk as far to the left as possible, at least until the eyes are looking fully to the rear (without turning the head). Keep the elbows pressed

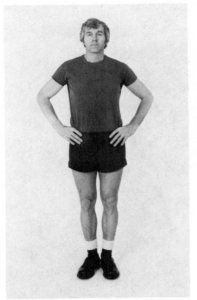

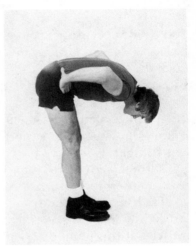

(Trunk Bending Fore and Aft)
Starting and finishing position

One

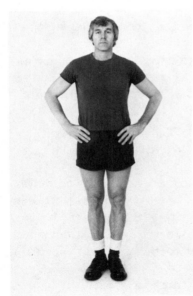

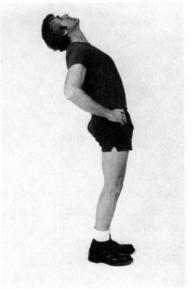

Two

Three

rearward and keep the feet firmly planted on the ground, pointing forward (your right foot may have a tendency to move).

TWO   Recover to the starting position with a clockwise twist of the trunk. Keep the elbows pressed rearward.

THREE   Twist the trunk as far to the right as possible, at least until the eyes are looking fully to the rear. Keep the elbows pressed rearward, the feet firmly planted.

FOUR   Recover to the starting position with a counterclockwise twist of the trunk. Check the elbows.

Comments • Resist any tendency for the elbows to sag forward or for the feet to move. Also resist any tendency to interlace the fingers behind the head, or to cup one hand over the other.

You are again stretching and strengthening those lower torso muscles; but note that you are doing this in a way that does not exactly duplicate the way you go about it with either the Side Twister Stretcher or the Trunk Rotation. Note also that you are involving the arms in different ways in these exercises. Because muscles are used in different combinations (and at different rhythms) in the athletic arena, they must also be used in different combinations in a truly comprehensive conditioning program.

7. Windmill, Four-Count

Starting Position • Standing at the position of attention, place the feet about three to three and a half feet apart. Extend the arms fully outward from the sides, parallel to the ground. Face the palms of the hands forward, with the fingers fully extended. Lock the elbows and the knees.

Execution • ONE   Simultaneously twisting the trunk counterclockwise and bending down at the waist, touch the left toes with the right fingertips. The left arm is now pointing straight upward, and the eyes are looking directly upward. (If at first you are unable to touch the toes, reach

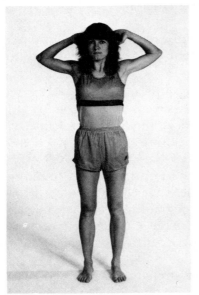

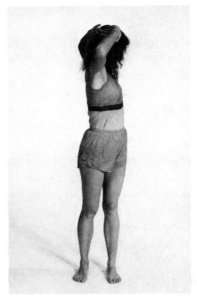

(Trunk Twister) Starting position

One

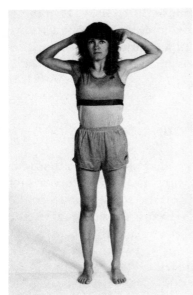

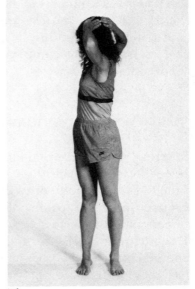

Two

Three

toward them.) You should feel a pulling sensation behind the knee area.

TWO   Recover to the starting position by reversing the ONE count: twist the trunk clockwise while simultaneously bending upward at the waist until the trunk is fully erect. Press the extended arms rearward while pushing the chest outward (you should feel a stretch in the upper arms, just above the armpits).

THREE   Simultaneously twisting the trunk clockwise and bending down at the waist, touch the right toes with the left fingertips. The right arm is now pointing straight upward; the eyes are looking directly upward.

FOUR   Recover to the starting position by reversing the THREE count: twist the trunk counterclockwise while simultaneously bending upward at the waist until the trunk is fully erect. Press the extended arms to the rear while pushing the chest outward.

Comments • Keep the arms fully extended and the elbows locked; also keep the knees locked. Pick up speed only as you become more proficient.

Work toward touching the ground beyond (to the far side of) the foot on the ONE and THREE counts.

The object here once again is to stretch muscles while simultaneously strengthening them—*and* to enhance overall athletic agility by requiring elements of coordination, rhythm, balance, and form. The reason most bodybuilders (weightlifters) usually are not particularly good athletes is because their muscles are strong only; that is, their muscles lack that flexibility and comprehensive, coordinated toning that is essential to general athletic competence.

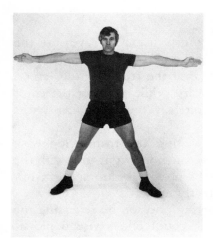

(Windmill, Four-Count) Starting and finishing position

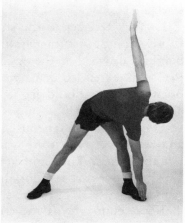

One

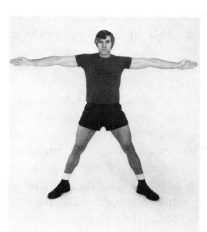

Two

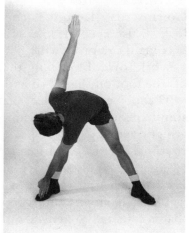

Three

8. Windmill, Two-Count

Starting Position • Standing at the position of attention, place the feet two to two and a half feet apart. With the knees firmly locked, bend deeply at the waist until the trunk is parallel to the ground. Extend the arms outward from the shoulders—parallel to the ground—and lock the elbows; face the palms toward the ground and extend the fingers.

Execution • ONE Twist the trunk vigorously leftward until the fingers of the extended right arm just touch the big toe of the left foot; reach for the ground beyond the foot. Simultaneously use the momentum of the rotating left arm to press that arm as far over the back as you can. The eyes are now looking directly leftward.

TWO Twist the trunk vigorously rightward until the fingers of the extended left arm just touch the big toe of the right foot; reach for the ground beyond the foot. Simultaneously use the momentum of the rotating right arm to press that arm as far over the back as you can. The eyes are now looking directly rightward.

Comments • Do not "reach" for your big toe; instead, twist the trunk until the fingers naturally touch it, then reach beyond the foot as far as you can. Keep the arms fully extended and the elbows firmly locked; also keep the knees firmly locked.

Avoid spreading the feet farther apart than the two to two and a half feet specified.

Increase the tempo until you are twisting back and forth as rapidly as possible without losing control of form.

Like the Half Jumping Jack, the Two-Count Windmill is an excellent exercise for getting the heart and lungs into high gear.

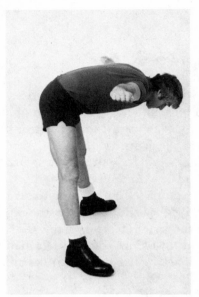 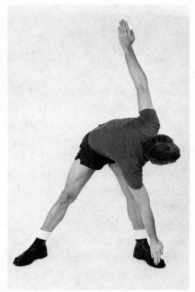

(Windmill, Two-Count) Starting position   One

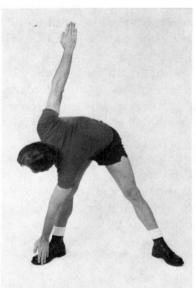

Two

9. Trunk Side Stretcher

Starting Position • Assume the starting position for the Trunk Twister, except place the feet together. The upper part of the fingers are against the back of the head, with the middle fingers just touching; the elbows are pressed rearward. The knees are locked.

Execution • ONE   Bending the trunk over the right hip, lean directly to the right as if to touch the right hip with the right elbow. Be sure to keep the fingers firmly planted against the back of the head, with the middle fingers just touching.

TWO   Recover to the starting position with a smooth leftward lift of the trunk. Check the position of the hands behind the head. Be sure the elbows are pressed rearward.

THREE   Bending the trunk over the left hip, lean directly to the left as if to touch the left hip with the left elbow. Be sure to keep the fingers firmly planted behind the head.

FOUR   Recover to the starting position with a smooth rightward lift of the trunk. Check the position of the hands behind the head. Keep the elbows pressed rearward.

Comments • Be conscious of keeping the fingers firmly planted against the back of the head, with the middle fingers just touching. Increase the tempo with proficiency.

A good exercise for melting away those "love handles."

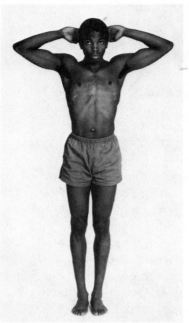

(Trunk Side Stretcher) Starting and finishing position

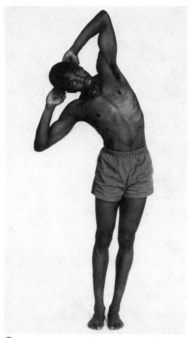

One

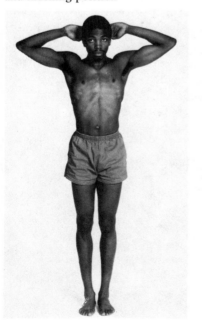

Two

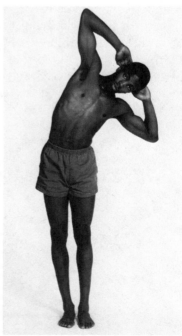

Three

10. Rocking Chair

Starting Position • Standing at the position of attention, place the feet comfortably apart, about three to four inches. Place the hands on the hips, fingers forward and thumbs rearward. Lock the knees.

Execution • ONE   Bending the trunk forward at the waist, reach down and touch the fingertips to the ground just in front of the toes (keeping the knees firmly locked). If at first you are unable to touch the ground, reach toward it. With the fingertips touching the ground (arms fully extended), lock the elbows.

TWO   Squat down fully by bending the knees until the buttocks are nearly resting on the heels (keeping the feet *flat* on the ground); simultaneously rotate the extended arms upward until they are parallel to the ground and extending directly forward. (The arms will tend to rotate upward as you squat down.) Be sure to keep the feet flat on the ground at all times; that is, do not roll up onto the balls of the feet.

THREE   Recover to the TWO-count position: straightening the legs, rotate the extended arms downward until the fingertips are once again touching the ground just in front of the toes. Lock the knees firmly.

FOUR   Recover to the starting position by lifting the trunk and placing the hands back on the hips.

Comments • Be sure to lock the knees at the end of the THREE count. Increase the tempo with proficiency. (Never sacrifice form to speed in this or any other exercise.)

Besides stretching and strengthening several important muscles in the legs, abdomen, back, and arms, the Rocking Chair will serve to enhance your coordination and balance skills (and therefore your overall athletic agility).

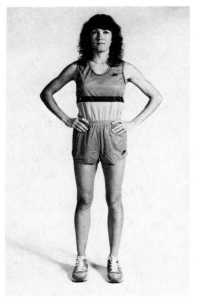

(Rocking Chair) Starting and finishing position

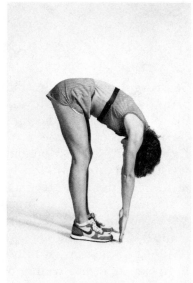

One

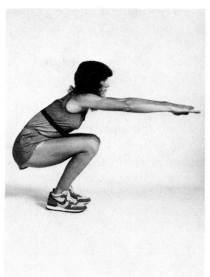

Two

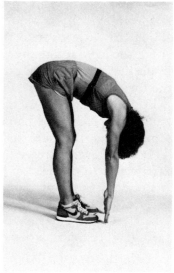

Three

The Abdominal Exercises

11. Regulation Sit-Up
12. Hand-and-Toe Sit-Up
13. Cherry Picker
14. Back Flutter Kick
15. Stomach Flutter Kick
16. Sitting Flutter Kick
17. Back Roller
18. Stomach Stretcher
19. Sitting Knee Bend
20. Leg Lever
21. Leg Thrust

The Abdominal Exercises are designed to stretch and strengthen the important muscles of the abdominal region: the extensor muscles of the lower back and the hips, the hip-joint flexors, the front trunk muscles, and the front thigh muscles. You may at first find some of these exercises difficult to perform—in particular, the Hand-and-Toe Sit-Up, the Flutter Kicks, and the Stomach Stretcher. Take each exercise step by step and stick with it until you get the hang of it. Keep in mind, however, that you do not need to perform some of these exercises until you are well into the formal exercise schedule.

As in the case of the General Warm-Up Exercises (and all the other exercises in the Calisthenics Program), the Abdominal Exercises are dynamic exercises that require you to move body mass through space, or to resist the force of gravity, often in ways that require coordination, flexibility, and balance. In doing this, the Abdominal Exercises not only strengthen the muscles involved; they also serve to enhance overall athletic agility.

Several of the Abdominal Exercises—notably the Flutter Kicks and the Leg Thrust—will test and ultimately enhance your physical and mental stamina as well.

11. Regulation Sit-Up

Starting Position • Lying prone on the back, place the hands against the back of the head, palms facing inward, fingers interlaced. Bend the knees until the knee joint is elevated about one foot off the ground. (As you gain proficiency with this exercise, gradually increase the elevation of the knees until they are as high off the ground as possible.) Squeeze the knees together with enough pressure to keep them together throughout the exercise. If you have a partner, have him or her bear down on your ankles with sufficient pressure to keep your heels firmly planted on the ground. Otherwise, you may want to hook the instep of the feet under some kind of unyielding restraint (for example, the bottom of a chest of drawers). Press the elbows rearward until the arms are in full contact with the ground.

Execution • ONE Bending at the waist, lift the trunk smoothy upward and touch the knees gently with the forehead. (If at first you are unable to touch the knees, reach toward them.) Keep the heels planted on the ground, the fingers interlaced behind the head.

TWO Recover to the starting position by *slowly* lowering the trunk backward. Pause in the prone position before beginning the ONE count of the next cycle; in other words, refrain from bouncing off the ground to take advantage of the momentum of recoil.

Comments • To be executed correctly, the Regulation Sit-Up should be executed slowly and deliberately, and with a strict adherence to proper form. Be conscious of keeping the fingers firmly interlaced behind the head and of keeping the heels or feet firmly planted on the ground.

As you become proficient, increase the elevation of the knees. This will greatly increase the effectiveness of the exercise. To get an idea of what this exercise does, pause when the trunk is at a forty-five degree angle relative to the ground and push in on the stomach with a finger. There is no better exercise for acquiring an "iron" stomach.

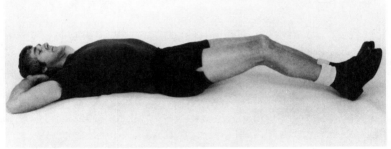

(Regulation Sit-Up) Starting
and finishing position

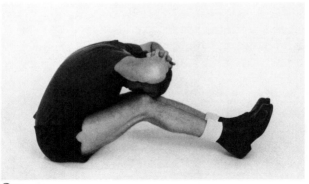

One

12. Hand-and-Toe Sit-Up

Starting Position • Lying prone on the back, extend the arms above the head and rest them on the ground; face the palms upward. Squeeze the legs snugly together and lock the knees.

Execution • ONE Simultaneously lifting the trunk and the legs, rotate the extended arms forward and touch the elevated toes. The legs are now at about a sixty-degree angle relative to the ground. (If at first you are unable to touch the toes, reach toward them.) *Keep the knees as rigidly locked as possible.*

TWO Recover to the starting point by slowly lowering the legs and the trunk to the ground, while simultaneously rotating the extended arms over the head to the ground.

Comments • The execution of this exercise should be smooth and controlled. However, because this exercise is not easy, it may take you a while to gain full control of it. Strive to keep the knees locked and to maintain your balance. Resist any tendency to pause after the TWO counts.

Inhale on the ONE count, exhale on the TWO count.

The Hand-and-Toe Sit-Up not only helps strengthen the abdominal muscles; it also enhances coordination and balance, and will test and ultimately enhance your mental as well as physical stamina. This exercise is most effective if you wear heavy boots (or ankle weights) while performing it.

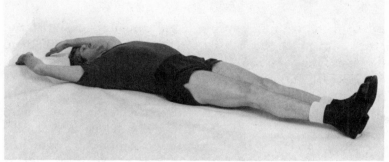

(Hand-and-Toe Sit-Up) Starting and finishing position

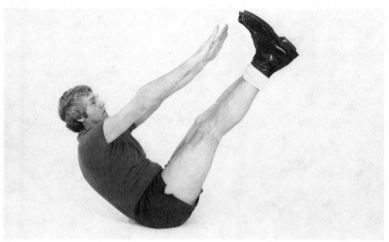

One

13. Cherry Picker

Starting Position • Standing at the position of attention,
place the feet three to four feet apart and place the hands on
the hips, fingers forward, thumbs rearward. Lock the knees
firmly.

Execution • ONE   Bending forward at the waist, reach
down and touch the palms of the hands on the ground.

   TWO   Lifting the trunk (no higher than parallel to the
ground), simultaneously cross the forearms one atop the

other; then, without pausing, bend down at the waist and attempt to touch the crossed forearms on the ground. Bend down as far as you can without losing your balance.

THREE   Lifting the trunk (no higher than parallel to the ground), simultaneously uncross the forearms; then, without pausing, bend down at the waist and touch the ground with the extended fingers as far back between the legs as you can.

FOUR   Recover to the starting position by lifting the trunk smoothly upward; place the hands back on the hips.

Comments • If on the ONE counts you are not able to touch the palms on the ground, reach down with the palms on each ONE count, using the fingertips as fulcrum points.

Be conscious of keeping the knees firmly locked. Increase the tempo with proficiency.

The Cherry Picker provides a good deal of redundant attention to those front trunk and lower back muscles. But, as you can readily feel, it also involves the groin and thigh muscles.

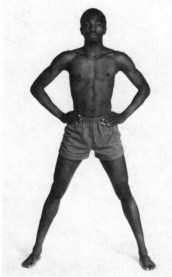

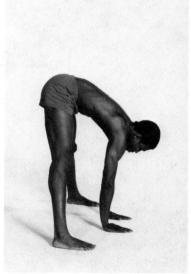

(Cherry Picker) Starting and   One
finishing position

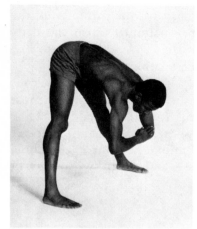

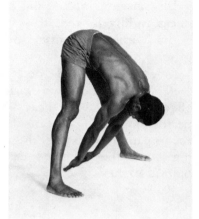

Two   Three

14. Back Flutter Kick

Starting Position • Lying prone on the back, place the hands, palms facing downward, under the hips; cushion the hipbones between the thumbs and the index fingers. Locking the knees, raise the rigid legs until the heels are one to two feet off the ground; point the toes away from the body. Raise the head three or four inches off the ground.

Execution • Alternately flutter the rigid legs up and down through an arc of two or three feet; move the legs from the hip joint only (that is, do not bend the knees at any time). Keep the knees firmly locked and the toes pointed. Keep a cycle count but not a step count. A cycle consists of the same leg moving up and down one time.

Comments • The Back Flutter Kick is a grueling but highly effective exercise. It is especially effective for strengthening the large abdominal and hip-joint flexor muscles, and is, therefore, of special value to runners, swimmers, divers, and iron-stomach enthusiasts.

Be conscious of keeping the head off the ground and the knees rigidly locked. If you are unable to finish the daily quota without a pause, lower the legs and head to the ground, count slowly to six, then resume the exercise.

Like the Hand-and-Toe Sit-Up, the Back Flutter Kick (as well as the other two varieties of Flutter Kick) is most effective if you wear heavy boots (or ankle weights) while performing it. The boots I'm wearing in the illustrations accompanying this exercise are military "jump" (parachuting) boots; they are size fourteens—and weigh two and a half pounds each!

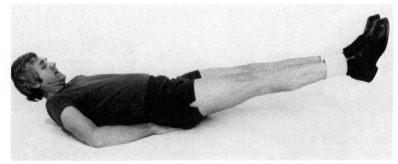

(Back Flutter Kick) Starting position

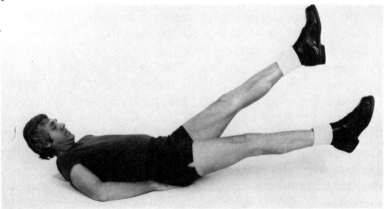

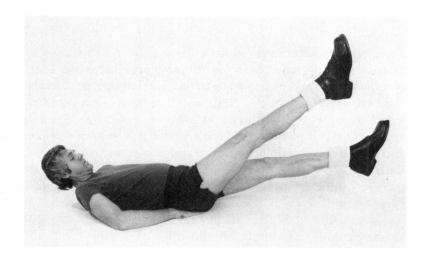

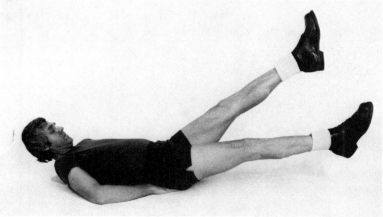

One

15. Stomach Flutter Kick

Starting Position • Lying prone on the stomach, extend the arms above the head and hold them elevated, parallel to the ground; face the palms toward the ground and lock the elbows. Lock the knees and lift the legs until the knees are no longer touching the ground; point the toes away from the body.

Execution • Alternately flutter the legs and arms up and down through the greatest possible arc, keeping the legs and arms as rigid as possible. Sustain a natural, coordinated rhythm, simultaneously elevating the right arm and leg while lowering the left arm and leg, and so forth. Keep a cycle count but not a step count. A cycle consists of the arm and leg on either side moving up and down one time.

Comments • The Stomach Flutter Kick is one of the least favorite among frogman and SEAL trainees. After a few cycles, you'll see why. Bear with this one.

The Stomach Flutter Kick is especially effective for strengthening and toning all the muscles of the back, the elevators and depressors of the arms, and the flexors and extensors of the hip joint.

Be conscious of keeping the arms and legs as rigid as possible. Try not to hold your breath.

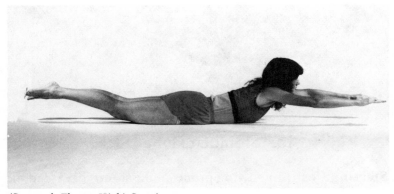

(Stomach Flutter Kick) Starting position

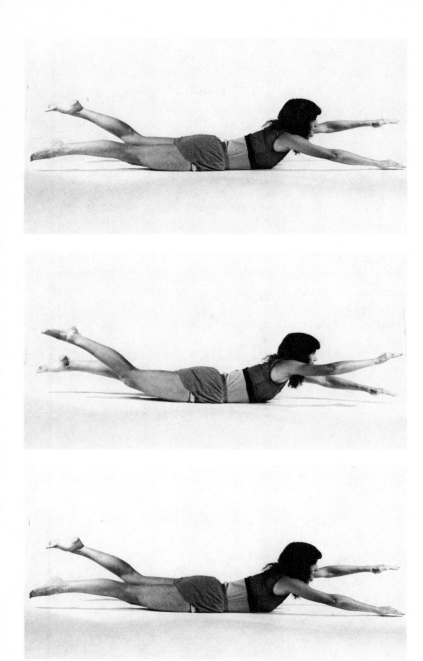

One

16. Sitting Flutter Kick

Starting Position • Assume a sitting position with the legs together and fully extended directly forward; lock the knees and point the toes away from the body. Place the right wrist over the left wrist and twist the wrists inward until the hands are palm to palm; interlock the fingers. Extend the arms over the head and squeeze the upper arms against the sides of the head. Lift the extended legs off the ground until the heels are elevated about one to one and a half feet. Maintain balance.

Execution • Alternately flutter the legs up and down through the greatest possible arc, keeping the legs as rigid as possible. Do not allow the heels to strike the ground. As with the other Flutter Kicks, keep a cycle count but not a step count. A cycle consists of the same leg moving up and down one time.

Comments • The Sitting Flutter Kick is another difficult but highly effective exercise. It is especially effective for strengthening and toning the abdominal and hip-joint flexor mus-

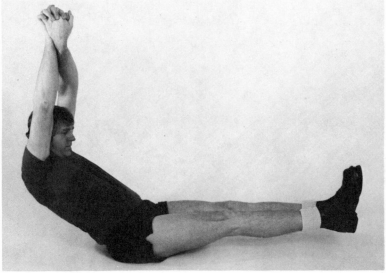

Starting position

cles—and for developing good coordination and balance. (It also serves to test your frustration and persistence levels!)

As with knocking your head against the wall, this exercise feels especially good when you stop. But bear with it; it's well worth the trouble.

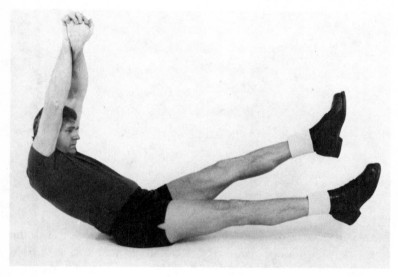

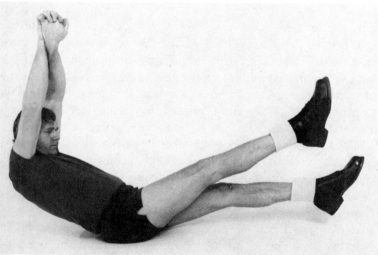

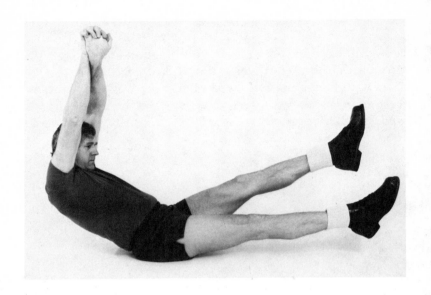

17. Back Roller

Starting Position • Lying prone on the back, extend the arms perpendicularly out from the sides; rest the extended arms on the ground, facing the palms downward. Lock the knees and squeeze the feet together with enough pressure to keep the legs together throughout the exercise. Elevate the rigid legs so that the heels are about six inches off the ground.

Execution • ONE Forcefully lifting the lower part of the body from the waist, rotate the legs over the body until the toes strike the ground above the head. The knees are now positioned just above the forehead, and your stern (to put it in nautical terms) is pointing toward the azure heavens.

TWO Recover to the starting position by rotating the legs back over the body; stop when the heels are about six inches from the ground. (*Do not* allow the heels to strike the ground.) Keep the head firmly on the ground throughout the count.

Comments • Keep the knees rigid, and keep the head and arms on the ground, at all times; *do not* allow the heels to strike the ground on the TWO count. Move as smoothly and continuously as possible.

At first, you may not be able to rotate the legs fully over the head. Keep trying.

Speed is not important with this exercise; concentrate on execution and form.

You can *feel* what the Back Roller is doing for your abdominal muscles at the end of the TWO counts, as you are "putting on the brakes" to prevent the heels from striking the ground.

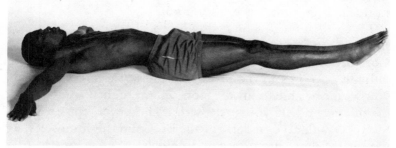

(Back Roller) Starting and finishing position

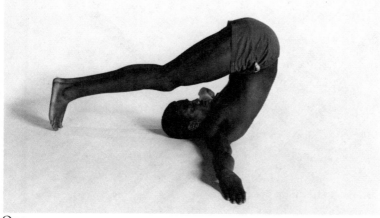

One

18. Stomach Stretcher

Starting Position • Lying prone on the back, bend the knees until the heels are nearly touching the buttocks, with the feet resting *flat* on the ground. Place the hands, palms facing downward, on the ground just above the shoulders, with the fingers pointing toward the tops of the shoulders; the elbows are now pointing upward.

Execution • ONE Arching the back, vigorously lift the stomach upward while allowing the head to drop backward until the eyes are looking parallel to the ground. Push the stomach as far into the air as you can.

TWO Ease the body slowly to the ground. Do not simply drop to the ground.

Comments • The Stomach Stretcher is one of the more difficult exercises in the program, and at first you may find you won't be able to lift the stomach more than a few inches off the ground. If you stick with it, however, the Stomach Stretcher will do wonders for the back and thigh muscles, as well as for those important abdominals.

Be persistent with this one.

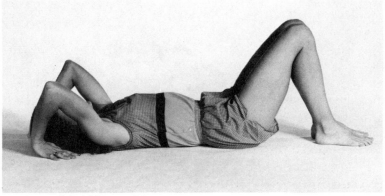

Starting and finishing position

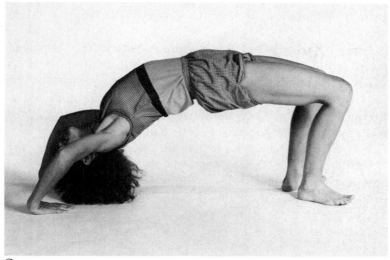

One

19. Sitting Knee Bend

Starting Position • Assume a sitting position with the legs together and extended directly forward; lock the knees. Place the right wrist over the left wrist and twist the wrists inward until the hands are palm to palm; interlock the fingers. Extend the arms over the head and squeeze the upper arms against the sides of the head. Elevate the extended legs until the heels are six inches off the ground. Maintain balance by leaning backward.

Execution • ONE Bending the knees, draw the feet smoothly inward and attempt to touch the groin area with the heels, without at any time allowing the feet to touch the ground. Maintain balance by leaning backward to the extent necessary.

TWO Recover to the starting position by smoothly straightening the legs, again without allowing the feet to touch the ground. Maintain balance.

Comments • You may at first have some difficulty maintaining balance, as your balance point changes as you move your legs. In time you will get the hang of it.

The Sitting Knee Bend is an excellent exercise for strengthening the abdominal muscles, the hip-joint flexor muscles, and the knee extensor muscles. It will also enhance your coordination and balance skills.

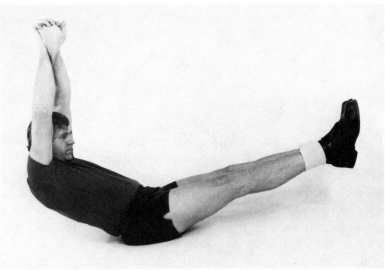

(Sitting Knee Bend) Starting
and finishing position

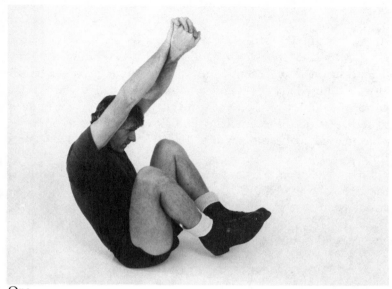

One

20. Leg Lever

Starting Position • Lying prone on the back, lock the knees and squeeze the feet together with enough pressure to keep the legs together throughout the exercise. If you have a partner, have your partner stand straddling your chest, facing your feet. Grab your partner's ankles. (If you do not have a partner, extend the arms out perpendicular to the sides and rest them on the ground.) Elevate the legs until the heels are six inches off the ground.

Execution • ONE   Lift the rigid legs and attempt to touch your partner (or an imaginary person straddling you) on the stomach.

   TWO   Have your partner catch your legs and push them away from himself. (If you do not have a partner, resist the upward motion of your legs, as if "putting on the brakes"; then lower your legs toward the ground.) Using a counterforce, prevent the heels from striking the ground.

Comments • The Leg Lever is an outstanding exercise for

strengthening the stomach muscles. (To see why, feel the
rigidity in the stomach during the TWO count.) In fact,
legend has it that Archie Moore, the famous boxer, person-
ally developed the Leg Lever (sometimes called the Archie
Moore) to build himself the kind of stomach he would need
to see his way to the title. (Legend also has it that no one ever
volunteered to be his partner for this exercise for a second
time.)

Note that the action of "putting on the brakes" to prevent
the heels from striking the ground at the end of the TWO
count is similar to the braking action you performed in the
Back Roller. Again, this exemplifies the kind of comprehensive redundancy that is built into this program.

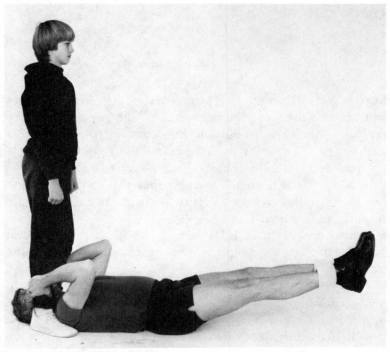

(Leg Lever) Starting and finishing position (with partner)

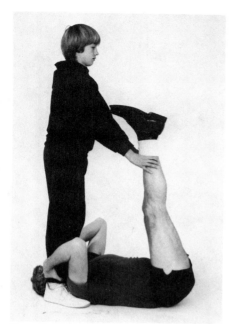

One

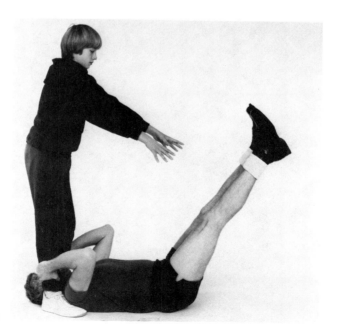

Two

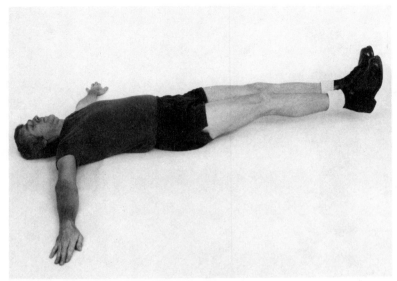

(Leg Lever) Starting and finishing position (without partner)

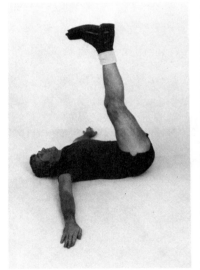

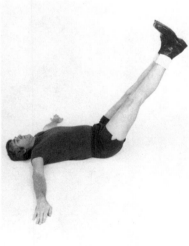

One

Two

21. Leg Thrust

Starting Position • Standing at the position of attention, squat down until you can place the hands flat on the ground, close together; do not squat down fully. Move the left foot forward and position it about three to four inches to the left of the left hand, with the toe tips in line with the fingertips. At the same time, extend the right leg as far to the rear as possible, resting it up on the ball of the foot. Face the toes of both feet forward; straighten the right leg. Lock the elbows.

Execution • ONE   Supporting the body weight with the arms, reverse the relative position of the legs by simultaneously thrusting the left foot rearward and the right foot forward. The left leg is now extended to the rear, resting up on the ball of the foot; the right foot is positioned three to four inches to the right of the right hand (with the toe tips in line with the fingertips).

TWO   Recover to the starting position by reversing the ONE count: simultaneously thrust the left foot forward and the right foot backward. The left leg is now positioned directly to the left of the left hand; the right leg is extended to the rear, resting up on the ball of the foot.

Comments • Fatigue is likely to overtake you quickly with this exercise, but maintain as rapid a pace as you can without losing control of form. Be conscious of bringing the toe tips all the way up in line with the fingertips, and of fully straightening the leg being thrust to the rear.

This is another one of those difficult exercises that are well worth mastering; keep at this one.

The Leg Thrust focuses on strengthening the hip and front thigh muscles, but involves muscles in many other areas as well, including the arms. The Leg Thrust is also an excellent stamina and coordination builder.

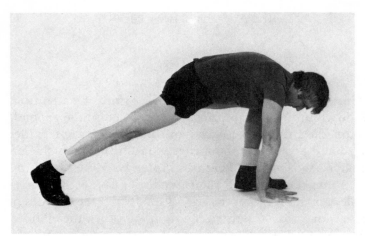

(Leg Thrust) Starting position

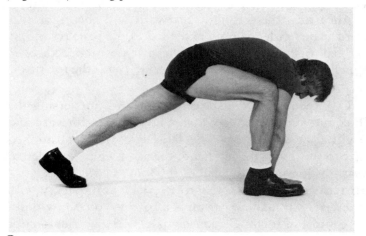

One

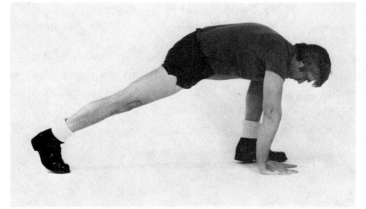

Two

The Side and Oblique Exercises

The Side and Oblique Exercises are designed to stretch and strengthen the important muscles that run obliquely over the back and chest, and those that run along the sides of the torso.

The first three exercises in this series require that you restrain either your shoulders or your legs by some means. If you have a partner, you can have him perform the required restraining; otherwise, you may have to rig some kind of restraining device. A wide belt secured to the ground or floor works very well.

22. Legs Flexing, Shoulders Secured

Starting Position • Lying prone on the stomach, rest the forehead comfortably on the hands; lock the knees with the legs pressed firmly together. Have your partner sit on your upper back (straddling you with his back toward your head works best), resting as much of his weight on you as you can bear. If you are using the belt restraint suggested at the beginning of this section, adjust the belt around your upper chest while lying on your back, then turn over.

Execution • ONE   Without bending the knees, use the rear thigh and lower back muscles to lift the legs, held as straight and firmly together as possible, as far up as possible; then allow them to ease downward, but do not allow them to touch the ground.

TWO   Repeat the ONE count.

THREE   Repeat the ONE count.

FOUR   Recover to the starting position by easing the legs to the ground. Do not simply drop the legs to the ground.

Comments • Maintain a slow, controlled pace; speed is not important here. Avoid thrusting the legs into the air if possible; instead, attempt to *lift* the legs, using the lower back and rear thigh muscles.

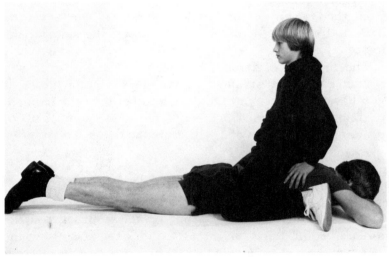

(Legs Flexing, Shoulders
Secured) Starting position

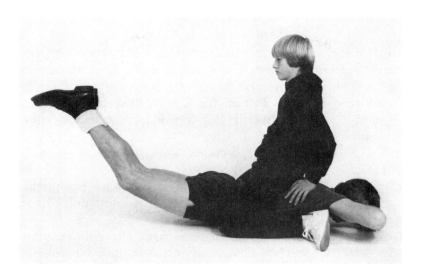

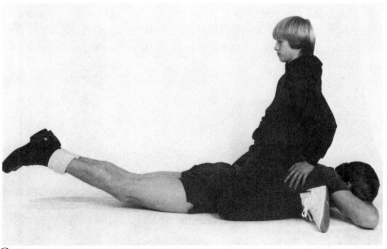

One

23. Back Flexing, Legs Secured

Starting Position • Lying prone on the stomach, extend the arms fully above the head and hold them elevated, parallel to the ground, palms facing downward. Have your partner sit on your legs, just below the knees (straddling the legs works best), and bear down with his full weight. Lock the knees and look directly forward.

Execution • ONE   Lift the trunk as far up as possible; then allow it to ease downward, but do not allow it to touch the ground.

TWO   Repeat the ONE count.

THREE   Repeat the ONE count.

FOUR   Recover to the starting position by easing the trunk to the ground. Do not simply drop the trunk to the ground.

Comments • If you do not have a partner to restrain your legs, use the wide-belt device suggested at the beginning of this section.

Maintain a slow, controlled pace. As with the Legs Flexing exercise, avoid thrusting the trunk into the air; instead, attempt to *lift* the trunk, using the back muscles. Note that extending the arms adds torque that must be overcome with greater effort.

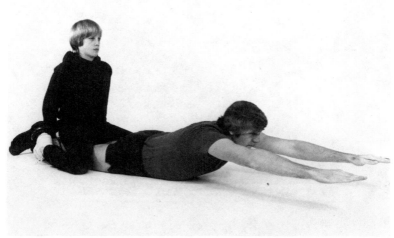

(Back Flexing, Legs Secured)
Starting and finishing position

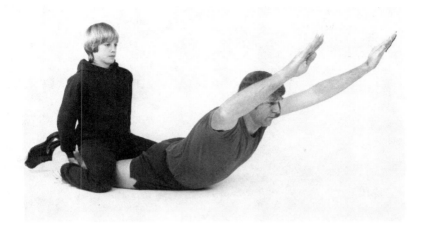

24. Side Flexing, Legs Secured

Starting Position • Lying prone on the left side, place the palms against the back of the head and interlace the fingers. Straighten the legs with the right leg atop the left leg, and lock the knees. Have your partner sit on your legs, straddling you so he can squeeze your legs together with his (to prevent your legs from slipping apart). Alternatively, restrain your legs with the wide belt suggested at the beginning of this section.

Execution • ONE   Lift the trunk as far over the right hip as possible. Attempt to touch the right side with the right elbow—without moving the hands from the back of the head.

TWO   Recover to the starting position by easing the trunk to the ground. Do not simply drop the trunk to the ground.

Comments • When halfway through the scheduled quota, roll onto the right side and complete the quota bending over the left side.

This exercise is difficult, but if you persist, you'll get the hang of it.

Side Flexing is an excellent exercise for strengthening the side muscles along the torso, but it also serves to enhance the flexibility of those muscles.

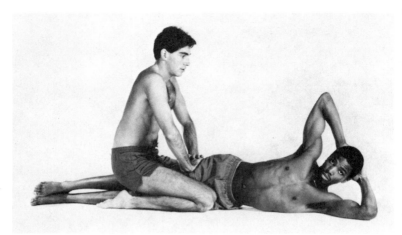

(Side Flexing, Legs Secured) Starting and finishing position

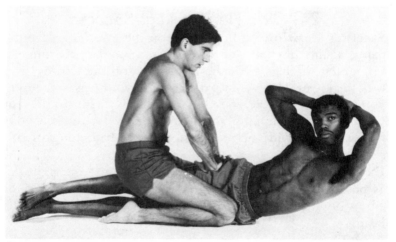

One

25. Sitting Back Bends

Starting Position • Assume a sitting position and spread the legs as far apart as possible; lock the knees. Place the hands against the forehead, palms facing outward, and interlace the fingers; press the elbows rearward. Straighten the head and trunk.

Execution • ONE Bend forward at the waist and touch the ground with the palms, without pulling the hands away from the forehead. If you are unable to touch the ground (and you probably will be) reach toward it.

TWO   Recover to the starting position by smoothly lifting the trunk. Keep the elbows pressed rearward.

Comments • At first (and perhaps for quite some time), you may not be able to touch the ground with your forehead. Keep trying. Gently.

The Sitting Back Bend is an excellent exercise for enhancing flexibility in those back muscles, but is equally valuable as a groin stretcher.

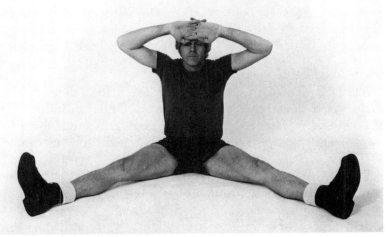

(Sitting Back Bends) Starting and finishing position

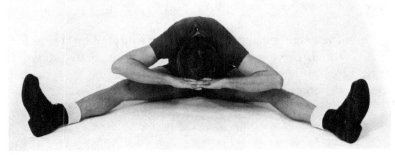

One

26. Side Snapper

Starting Position • Standing at the position of attention, place the feet comfortably apart, about one and a half to two feet; lock the knees. Extend the arms out from the sides, parallel to the ground, with the palms facing downward. Keep the head up.

Execution • ONE   Bend the trunk sideways to the right until the fingers of the extended right arm touch as far down the right leg as possible; simultaneously relax the left arm and allow it to bend (snap) loosely over the head. The left fingers should strike the top of the head.

TWO   Recover to the starting position by lifting the trunk leftward and simultaneously re-extending the left arm out from the side.

THREE   Bend the trunk sideways to the left until the fingers of the extended left arm touch as far down the left leg as possible; simultaneously relax the right arm and allow it to bend (snap) loosely over the head. The right fingers should strike the top of the head.

FOUR   Recover to the starting position by lifting the trunk rightward and simultaneously re-extending the right arm out from the side.

Comments • In addition to stretching and strengthening the muscles along the torso, the Side Snapper will help develop your coordination skills. (This is one of those exercises you may want to practice before you begin the program in earnest.)

Keep the extended arm straight; that is, avoid lowering the arm to touch the leg instead of bending the torso sideways until the extended arm comes in contact with the leg (you can feel the difference).

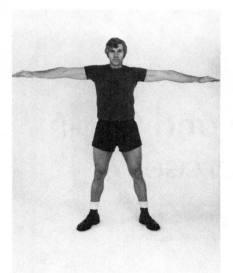

(Side Snapper) Starting and
finishing position

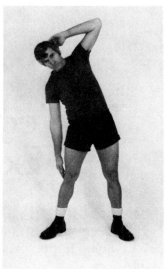

One

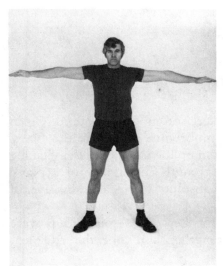

Two

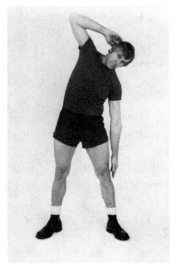

Three

The Leg and Groin Exercises

The large number of exercises in the Leg and Groin category reflects the high importance placed by the Navy special forces training program on the muscles in the vital leg area. Needless to say, the strength and agility of a Navy frogman or SEAL's legs are absolutely critical to his overall mission.

The twelve exercises in the Leg and Groin group were specifically designed to strengthen and tone the vital leg, knee, and groin muscles.

27. Deep Knee Bender, Four-Count

Starting Position • Standing at the position of attention, place the hands on the hips, fingers forward, thumbs rearward. Keep the head up, eyes forward.

Execution • ONE   Keeping the trunk straight, bend the knees until you are in a half-squat position; that is, until the knees are about fourteen to eighteen inches forward. *Do not* squat down fully. Simultaneously extend both arms forward and hold them parallel to the ground, palms downward. Come to a full stop before executing the TWO count.

TWO   Keeping the feet *flat* on the ground, bend the knees until you are in a full-squat position; keep the extended arms parallel to the ground, the back straight. *Do not* roll up onto the balls of the feet.

THREE   Lift yourself to the ONE-count position by partially straightening the legs. Come to a complete stop, with the knees partially bent, the arms fully extended forward.

FOUR   Recover to the starting position by fully straightening the legs and placing the hands back on the hips.

Comments • The Four-Count Deep Knee Bender is an excellent leg and knee-area strengthener, provided you pay strict attention to proper execution. Keep the back straight, keep the feet flat on the ground at all times, and come to a complete stop at the end of each count. The extended arms will help you maintain balance.

Maintain a slow, controlled pace.

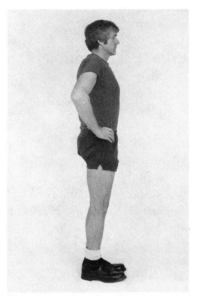

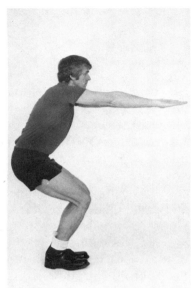

(Deep Knee Bender, Four-Count) Starting and finishing position

One

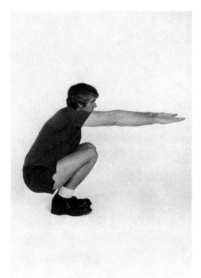

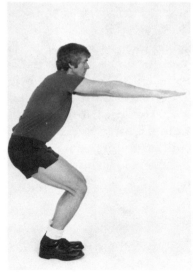

Two

Three

28. Deep Knee Bender, Two-Count

Starting Position • Same as for the Four-Count Deep Knee Bender.

Execution • ONE   Keeping the feet *flat* on the ground, bend the knees until you are *fully* squatting; simultaneously extend the arms forward and hold them parallel to the ground. Keep the back straight. Come to a full stop; that is, do not bounce off the low point.

TWO   Recover to the starting position by fully straightening the legs and placing the hands back on the hips.

Comments • Maintain as rapid a pace as you can without losing control of execution and form. Keep the feet flat on the ground as you squat, and keep the back straight. Consciously pause at the end of the ONE count.

In addition to helping strengthen the legs and the knee area, the Two-Count Deep Knee Bender will help enhance coordination, balance, and stamina.

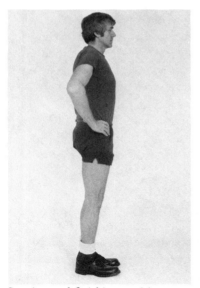
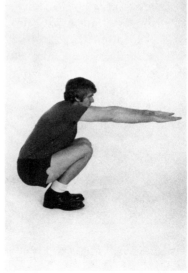

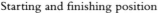
Starting and finishing position   One

29. Squat Jump

Starting Position • Assume a squat-kneel position; that is, squat down fully, then, keeping the left foot *flat* on the ground, move the right foot rearward until the thigh is parallel to the ground and the knee is pointing directly forward. The right foot is now resting up on the ball of the foot with the right buttock resting on the heel. Place the palms against the back of the head and interlace the fingers; press the elbows rearward. Straighten the back and keep the head up.

Execution • ONE　Springing upward, quickly reverse the relative positions of the legs by simultaneously moving the left foot rearward, the right foot forward. Maintain balance.

　　TWO　Recover to the starting position by springing upward and quickly shifting the relative positions of the legs.

Comments • The Squat Jump is not an easy exercise, but it is an *outstanding* exercise for strengthening the leg muscles. (Your legs will tell you this in short order!) It is also an excellent exercise for sharpening your coordination. Endure this one by thinking about all the good it is doing you.

　　If you intend to play basketball and wish to enhance your rebounding proficiency, you may want to do a few Squat Jumps every day instead of only when they are formally scheduled. (Also see the Squat Stretch.)

　　Increase the tempo with proficiency. Keep the back straight and the fingers firmly interlaced behind the head.

30. Leg Stretcher

Starting Position • Assume a sitting position with the right leg doubled backward (alongside, not under, the body) so that the right heel rests against the right hip. (This contortion may be a little uncomfortable at first, until your muscles stretch out.) Extend the left leg and spread it as far to the left

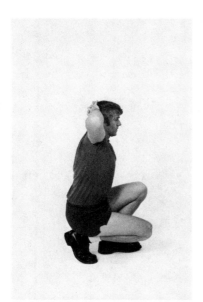

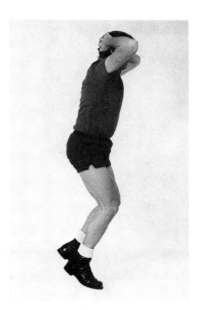

(Squat Jump) Starting and
finishing position

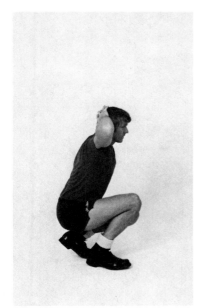

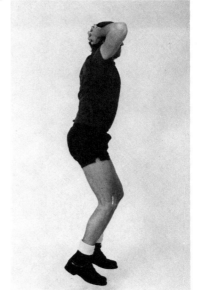

One

as you can; point the toes directly upward and lock the knee. Place the palms against the back of the head and interlace the fingers; press the elbows rearward. Straighten the trunk.

Execution • ONE   Bending forward at the waist, attempt to touch the left knee with the forehead. If you are unable to touch the knee, reach toward it. Gently. Keep the knee locked.

TWO   Lift the trunk smoothly to the starting position, then lean directly backward until you feel the muscles in the right thigh stretching.

Comments • The Leg Stretcher can be rather uncomfortable at first. But if you bear with it, in time those reluctant muscles will stretch out. Be conscious of keeping the toes of the extended leg pointed upward, and of keeping the knee of that leg as rigidly locked as possible. Speed is not important here; concentrate on execution and form.

Halfway through the scheduled quota, reverse the relative positions of the legs and attempt to touch the right knee with the forehead.

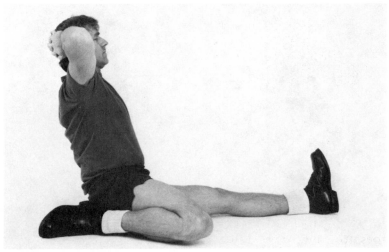

(Leg Stretcher) Starting position

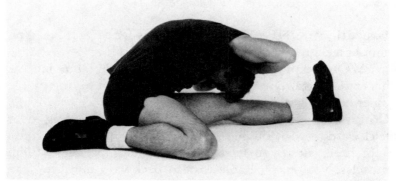

One

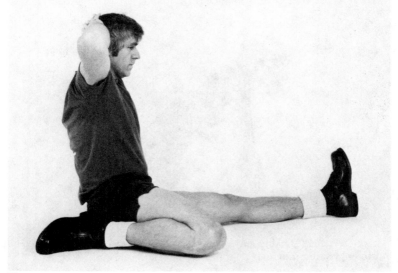

Two

31. Thigh Stretcher

Starting Position • Assume a kneeling position with the knees together, buttocks resting on the heels. Keeping the toes together, spread the heels apart and lean backward, using the arms for support. Lean backward at least until you are looking directly upward—further backward if you can.

Execution • ONE Lift the hips up as far as possible. You should feel the muscles in the thighs stretching.

TWO Recover to the starting position by allowing the hips to sink gently until the buttocks are again resting on the inner heels. (Keep the heels spread as far apart as possible.)

Comments • This exercise will have you bending over backward (sorry, couldn't resist).

In time, after you have stretched out those tight thigh muscles, you may be able to lean backward until you can actually touch the ground with the back of your head.

Bear with this one; it's worth it.

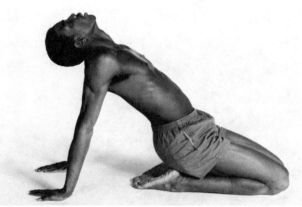

(Thigh Stretcher) Starting and finishing position (normal)

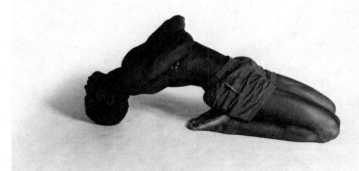

Starting and finishing position (goal)

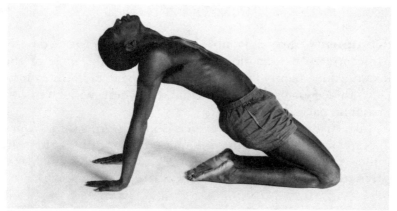

One

32. Groin Stretcher, Four-Count

Starting Position • Standing at the position of attention, spread the legs widely apart, about three to four feet. Cross the forearms with the palms atop the elbows (Indian style); extend the upper arms directly forward so that the forearms are parallel to the ground. Straighten the back; lock the knees.

Execution • ONE Keeping the right knee locked, bend the left knee fully while rotating the upper body slightly to the right; allow the body to sink down and rest fully on the folded left leg. You are now fully squatting on the left leg, with the right leg extending fully out to the right and resting on the heel of the foot. You should feel the muscles under the right thigh being "asked" to stretch out. Keep the folded forearms out from the chest.

TWO Recover to the starting position by straightening the left leg while rotating the upper body slightly to the left.

THREE Keeping the left knee locked, bend the right knee fully while rotating the upper body slightly to the left; allow the body to sink down and rest fully on the folded right leg.

FOUR Recover to the starting position by straightening the right leg while rotating the upper body slightly to the right.

Comments • Speed is not important with this exercise; concentrate on execution and form. Keep the knee of the extended leg firmly locked on the ONE and THREE counts. The folded arms held out from the chest will help you maintain balance.

Like many of the other exercises in this group, the Four-Count Groin Stretcher may be a bit uncomfortable at first. In time, though, the groin muscles will stretch out and strengthen, and the discomfort will largely disappear.

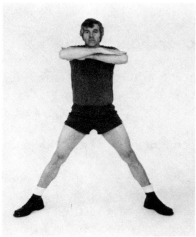

(Groin Stretcher, Four-Count)
Starting and finishing position

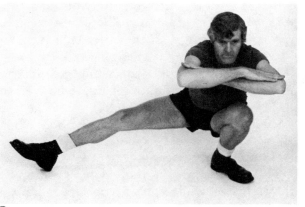

One

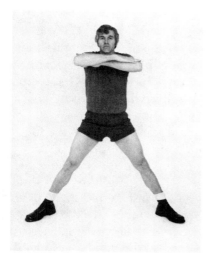

Two

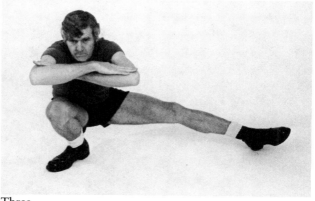

Three

33. Groin Stretcher, Two-Count

Starting Position • Assume the ONE-count position of the Four-Count Groin Stretcher: fully squat on the left leg with the right leg extending out to the right and resting on the heel of the foot; lock the right knee and hold the crossed forearms out from the chest.

Execution • ONE Lifting the body slightly with the left leg, shift the upper body rightward by fully extending the left leg while fully bending the right leg; do not raise the body all the way up to the starting position of the Four-Count Groin Stretcher. You are now in the THREE-count position of the Four-Count Groin Stretcher; that is, you are fully squatting on the right leg, with the left leg fully extended out to the left and resting up on the heel of the foot. The crossed forearms are extended out from the chest.

TWO   Recover to the starting position by reversing the ONE count: lift the body slightly with the right leg and shift the upper body leftward until you are fully squatting on the left leg again, with the right leg fully extended to the right.

Comments • You may at first tend to lose your balance as you shift your weight back and forth. Don't be discouraged if you do; this is a common experience with this exercise. Use the crossed forearms held out from the chest to help you keep your balance. Keep the extended leg firmly locked; squat fully.

Increase the tempo with proficiency.

In addition to helping stretch and strengthen those groin muscles, the Two-Count Groin Stretcher will do much to enhance your athletic agility.

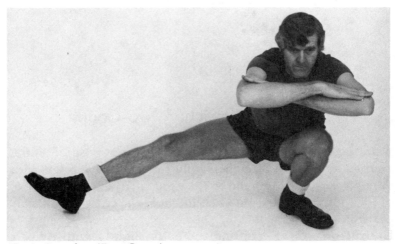

(Groin Stretcher, Two-Count)
Starting and finishing position

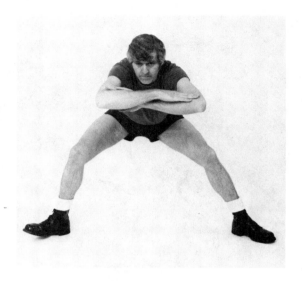

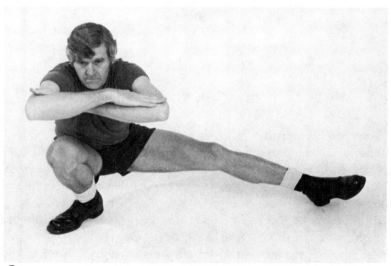

One

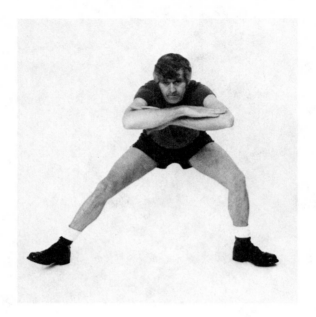

34. Calf Stretcher

Starting Position • Assume a sitting position with the legs extended and pressed together; lock the knees. Reach forward and grasp the toes of both feet. (At first, you may feel considerable resistance in the general knee area.) Keep the knees locked.

Execution • ONE Keeping the knees locked, pull the heels as far off the ground as you can. Gently.

TWO Recover to the starting position by allowing the heels to ease to the ground.

Comments • The Calf Stretcher can be rather uncomfortable the first few times you attempt it. Go at it gently—but persistently—and in time those important muscles around the knee will stretch out and strengthen, and the discomfort will largely disappear.

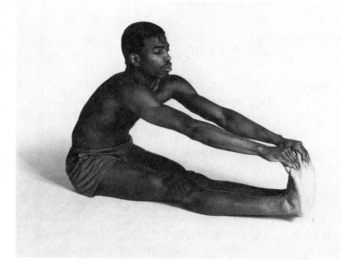

(Calf Stretcher) Starting and
finishing position

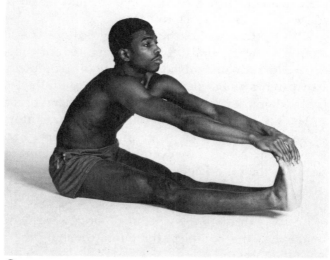

One

35. One-Legged Sit-Up

Starting Position • Assume the starting position for the Leg Stretcher, except extend the left leg directly forward instead of to the left. The right leg is doubled backward (alongside, not under, the body), with the heel resting against the right hip. Place the palms against the back of the head and interlace the fingers; press the elbows rearward. Now lean backward until the head and back are resting on the ground; if necessary, allow the knee of the doubled leg to rise. (You may have considerable difficulty leaning all the way back at first; keep trying.)

Execution • ONE   In the manner of the Regulation Sit-Up, lift the trunk smoothly upward and forward and touch the left knee with the forehead. Keep the left leg straight, the knee firmly locked; keep the hands behind the head. If unable to touch the knee, reach toward it.

TWO   Recover to the starting position by easing the trunk to the ground. Avoid rolling to one side to avoid discomfort in the doubled leg; come to a complete stop.

Comments • If at first you are unable to lift the trunk on the ONE count, keep trying; you'll get the hang of it in time.

The One-Legged Sit-Up can be a bit uncomfortable until those tight thigh and groin muscles begin to stretch and strengthen. Note, however, that you are not required to perform the One-Legged Sit-Up until the fifth week of the program—that is, after some of the easier exercises in the program have begun the stretching-out process.

Halfway through the scheduled quota, reverse the position of the legs and complete the quota touching the right knee with the forehead.

The One-Legged Sit-Up focuses on the thigh and groin muscles, but it also involves the abdominal muscles, and in a way similar to the way the Regulation Sit-Up involves the abdominal muscles. This is yet another example of the redundancy built into this program.

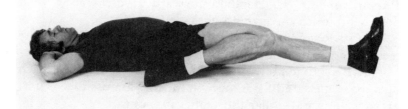

(One-Legged Sit-Up) Starting
and finishing position

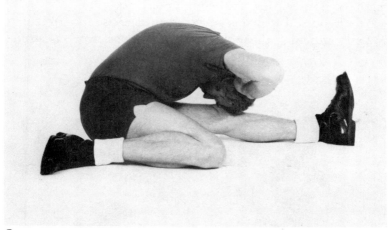

One

36. Bend and Reach

Starting Position • Standing at the position of attention,
place the feet about two inches apart and place the hands on

the hips, fingers forward, thumbs rearward. Lock the knees.

Execution • ONE   Bending forward at the waist, reach down and touch the ground with clenched fists.

TWO   Recover to the starting position by lifting the trunk and placing the hands back on the hips.

THREE   Extending the arms directly overhead, reach upward while standing as high on the toes as possible, as if to grasp a thousand-dollar bill that is just out of reach. Pause, maintaining balance.

FOUR   Recover to the starting position by lowering the arms and heels.

Comments • Stand as high up on the toes as you possibly can; consciously pause at the high point.

The Bend and Reach is an excellent exercise for stretching and strengthening those thigh and calf muscles. You can *feel* it!

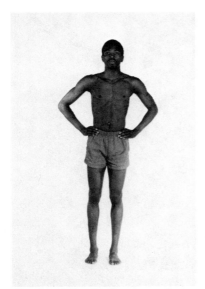

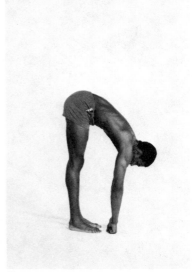

(Bend and Reach) Starting and   One
finishing position

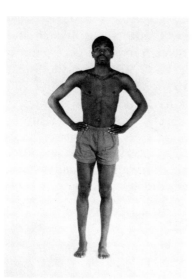

Two

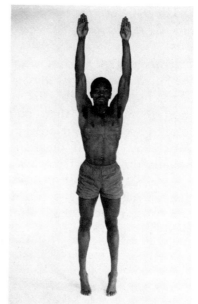

Three

37. Squat Stretch

Starting Position • Assume the squat-kneel starting position as for the Squat Jump.

Execution • ONE Jump vigorously upward (the feet should clear the ground by at least two feet), pushing the chest outward and upward to enhance your upward motion; simultaneously reverse the relative positions of the legs by shifting the left foot to the rear, the right foot forward. At the end of the count you are in a squat-kneel position with the right foot forward, resting flat on the ground, and with the left foot to the rear, resting up on the ball of the foot, with the left buttock resting on the heel. The back is straight and the fingers are firmly interlaced behind the head; the elbows are pressed rearward.

TWO   Recover to the starting position by jumping vigorously upward and reversing the relative positions of the legs.

Comments • The difference between the Squat Stretch and the Squat Jump is that the Squat Stretch requires you to jump to the highest possible extent on the ONE count; the Squat Jump requires only that you jump high enough to allow you time to reverse the relative positions of the legs.

Be conscious of pushing your chest out as you jump; literally throw yourself upward.

This is an exhausting exercise, but it gives back far more than it requires. The Squat Stretch is an especially good exercise for the basketball player, and for anyone else who needs springs for legs.

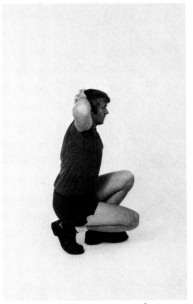
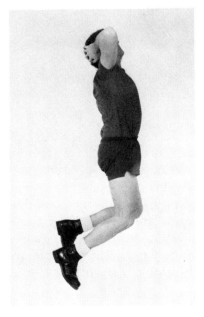

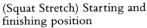
(Squat Stretch) Starting and finishing position

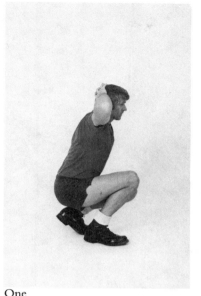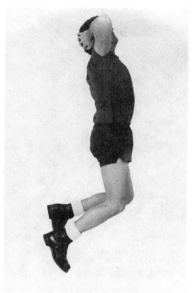

One

38. Good Morning Darling

Starting Position • Assume the prone starting position for the Back Flutter Kick. Be sure the knees are firmly locked and the toes are pointed outward, away from the body.

Execution • ONE   Spread the legs as far apart as possible, keeping them elevated. (At no point should the heels touch the ground.)

TWO   Recover to the starting position by closing the legs. Again, keep the legs elevated.

Comments • Keep the head and heels off the ground at all times. You may tire rapidly, but keep going. Maintain a rapid tempo, but not at the expense of failing to spread the legs fully on the ONE counts.

Besides providing redundant attention to the abdominal area, the Good Morning Darling serves to stretch and strengthen those groin flexors. An excellent exercise for swimmers who use the frog kick a lot (as I do).

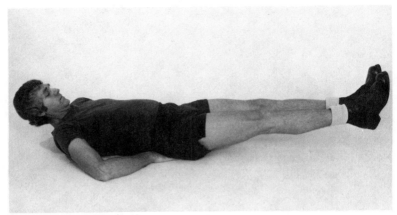

(Good Morning Darling)
Starting and finishing position

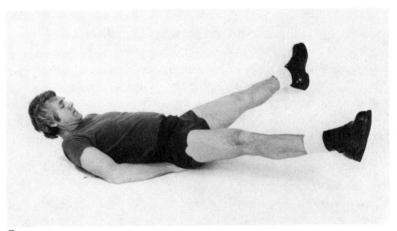

One

The Arm, Chest, and Shoulder Exercises

The Arm, Chest, and Shoulder Exercises are designed to stretch and strengthen the upper back muscles, the massive chest and shoulder muscles, and the important arm muscles. Though there are eight exercises listed in this group, there are effectively eleven exercises, because the Eight-Count Body Builder is essentially four exercises in one. (Keep this in mind when you're only halfway through the scheduled quota for the Eight-Count Body Builder—and about to fall flat on your face.)

To execute the Pull-Up, you will need a pull-up bar or an alternative device that can serve as one. You can make a pull-up bar out of a three- to four-foot length of one-inch pipe. Support the pipe in a level position about eight to nine feet off the ground. Make sure the bar as secured will support your full body weight. Possible alternatives to a bar include a rafter in the garage or the top of a nearby high fence.

39. Spread Eagle

Starting Position • Lying prone on the stomach, legs together, extend the arms above the head and rest them on the ground, palms facing downward. Lock the elbows and the knees.

Execution • ONE   Arching the back, lift the legs and arms as far off the ground as possible, *without bending either the knees or the elbows*.

TWO   Spreading the legs as far apart and upward as possible, simultaneously sweep the arms backward and upward until they are extended out from the shoulders and elevated as far as possible (poised like the wings of a gliding eagle). The palms are still facing downward. Keep the legs off the ground.

THREE   Recover to the ONE-count position by closing the legs and simultaneously moving the arms forward and downward until they are once again extended directly above the head (but not touching the ground).

FOUR   Ease the legs and arms gently to the ground. Do not simply drop them down.

Comments • Keep the palms facing downward at all times, and come to a full stop at the end of each count. Lift the arms and legs as far up as possible on the TWO counts.

The Spread Eagle provides redundant attention to the lower back and rear thighs, but the emphasis is on the upper arms and the shoulders. You'll feel this during the TWO counts.

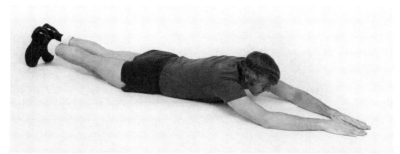

(Spread Eagle) Starting and
finishing position

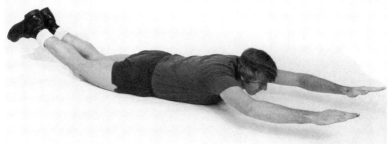

One

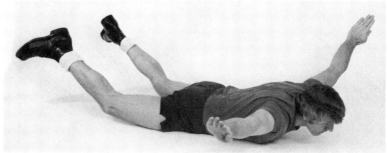

Two

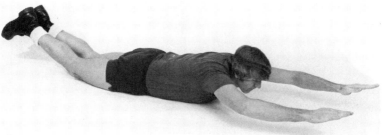

Three

40. Deep Breather

Starting Position • Standing at the position of attention, place the feet comfortably apart (a few inches) and place the hands on the hips, fingers forward, thumbs rearward. Hold in the stomach; stand tall.

Execution • ONE   Breathe in deeply, allowing only the chest to expand; that is, do not allow the abdomen to expand. Pause a moment.

TWO   Exhale, slowly; then pause a moment.

Comments • It is important to breathe slowly here, to prevent bringing on dizziness due to hyperventilation. Pause consciously at the end of each count.

Forcibly expand the chest cavity as much as possible on the ONE counts.

The Deep Breather serves to strengthen the diaphragm.

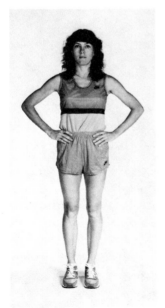 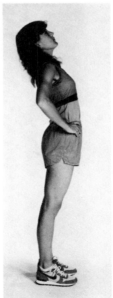 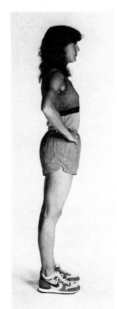

Starting position   One   Two

41. Eight-Count Body Builder

Starting Position • Standing at the position of attention, place the hands on the hips, fingers forward, thumbs rearward.

Execution • ONE   Squat fully, rolling up onto the balls of the feet, and place the palms on the ground about ten to twelve inches forward of, and slightly out from, the toes; lock the elbows. Keep the knees together.

TWO   Shifting the full body weight to the arms, thrust the legs fully to the rear; straighten the back and lock the knees.

THREE   Bending the elbows, allow the trunk to sink slowly until the nose just touches the ground. Pause, supporting your full weight. Keep the knees locked, the back straight. Do not allow your weight to rest on the ground.

FOUR   Recover to the TWO-count position by slowly straightening the arms; lock the elbows when the arms are fully extended.

FIVE   Thrusting the legs outward, spread the feet as far apart as possible; keep the knees locked, the back straight. (You may wish to add a step at this point, by doing a push-up while the legs are spread.)

SIX   Recover to the FOUR-count position by thrusting the legs inward.

SEVEN   Recover to the ONE-count position by thrusting the feet forward. You are now in a full-squat position, resting up on the balls of the feet.

EIGHT   Recover to the starting position by straightening the legs and placing the hands back on the hips.

Comments • The Eight-Count Body Builder is an outstanding exercise that will more than live up to its name, provided you give it your all, and provided you pay strict attention to form and execution. Increase the pace with proficiency.

Be conscious of keeping your back straight.

Though the Eight-Count Body Builder focuses on the arms and chest, it clearly involves several other areas, including the abdominal and groin areas.

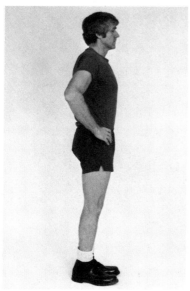

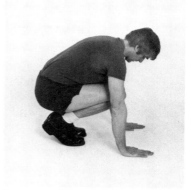

(Eight-Count Body Builder)
Starting and finishing position

One

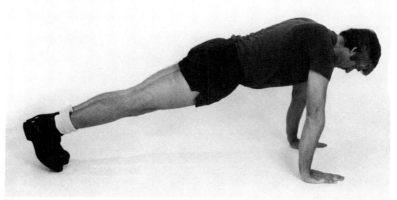

Two

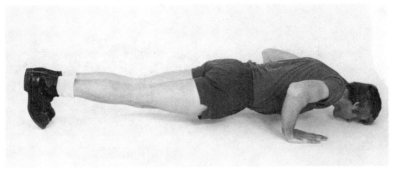

Three

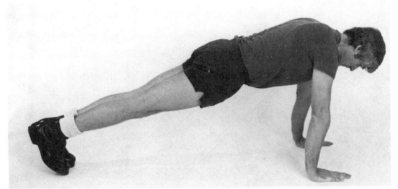

Four

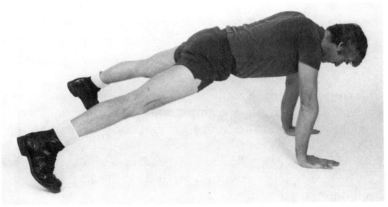

Five

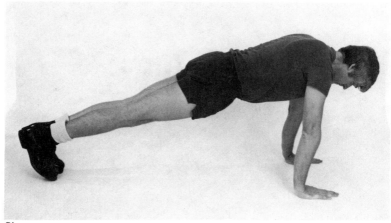

Six

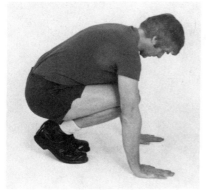

Seven

42. Neck Rotation

Starting Position • Standing at the position of attention, place the hands on the hips, fingers forward, thumbs rearward, and nod the head fully forward (without slumping).

Execution • ONE Rotate the head in a clockwise direction one complete revolution around the neck; pressing the head downward at all times.

Comments • Not too tough (a welcome interlude after the Eight-Count Body Builder), but important for neck muscle flexibility, especially for swimmers. When halfway through the day's quota, reverse the direction of rotation.

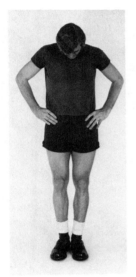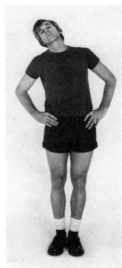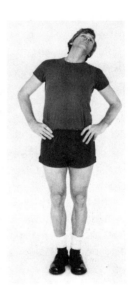

(Neck Rotation)
Starting and finishing
position

43. One-Legged Push-Ups

Starting Position • Assume the TWO-count position of the Eight-Count Body Builder (which is the starting position for the common push-up). Place the right foot atop the left heel so that only the left foot (ball of the left foot) is resting on the ground.

Execution • ONE   Bending the elbows, allow the trunk to sink slowly until the nose just touches the ground. Pause, supporting your full weight; do not allow your weight to rest on the ground. Keep the back straight.

TWO   Recover to the starting position by straightening the arms; lock the elbows when the arms are fully extended.

Comments • Be conscious of form and execution. Most push-ups are done incorrectly and therefore ineffectively. The most common errors are: moving the abdomen up and down instead of the entire trunk; bouncing off the ground to capitalize on the momentum of recoil; arching the back; failing to lower the nose fully to the ground on the ONE counts; failing to straighten the arms fully on the TWO counts. If you "cheat" on the One-Legged Push-Up, you of course only cheat good ol' Guess Who.

Halfway through the scheduled quota, reverse the relative position of the legs.

The attention to the arms and chest here is similar to that provided by the Eight-Count Body Builder; but the one-legged aspect of this exercise adds an extra element of balance and coordination.

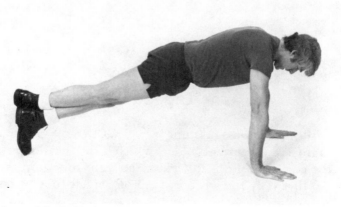

(One-Legged Push-Ups)
Starting and finishing position

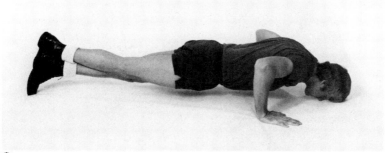

One

44. Press Press Fling

Starting Position • Standing at the position of attention, place the feet comfortably apart, about three or four inches, and extend the arms directly out from the chest; face the palms downward. Straighten the back.

Execution • PRESS   Bending the elbows, draw the open hands, thumbs first, smoothly toward the chest and attempt to touch the chest at the armpits. (You will not be able to actually touch the armpits.) Allowing the arms to recoil, move them back to the starting position.

PRESS   Repeat the previous count.

FLING   Pull the arms open and fling them as far to the rear as possible; simultaneously rotate the forearms so that the palms end up facing forward. Thrust the chest outward. Allowing the arms to recoil, return them to the starting position.

Comments • Maintain a lively pace. Stretch the arms as far to the rear as possible on the FLING count.

Note that the action during the FLING count is similar to (but again, not exactly like) the action of the arms at the end of the TWO count of the Four-Count Windmill—more built-in redundancy and comprehensiveness.

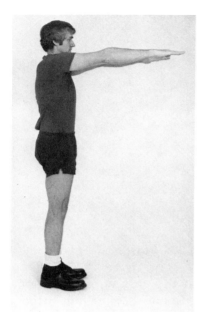
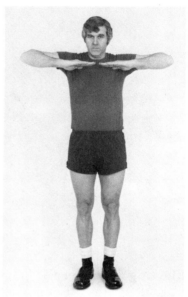

(Press Press Fling) Starting
position

Press

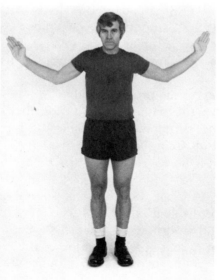

Fling

45. Up Back and Over

Starting Position • Standing at the position of attention, place the feet comfortably apart, about three or four inches, and extend the fingers fully at the sides.

Execution • UP Rotate the arms directly forward until fully extended over the head.

BACK Rotate the arms briskly downward, allowing them to swing slightly to the rear.

OVER Rotate the arms vigorously forward, then full circle over the head; allow the momentum of rotation to carry the arms toward the ONE count of the next cycle.

Comments • You will not be able to rotate your arms in a perfect circle on the OVER count. However, to cause your muscles to stretch to the maximum degree, you should strive to make the circle as nearly perfect as you can.

The Up Back and Over serves to enhance flexibility in the upper arms and the shoulders.

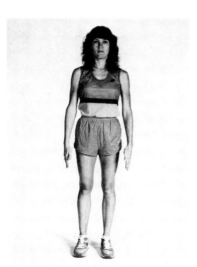

Starting position

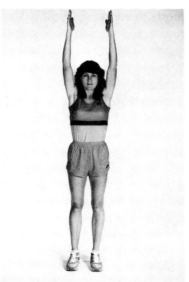

Up

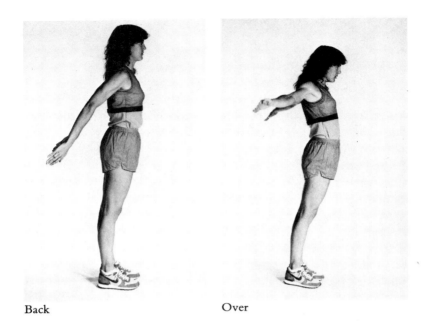

Back   Over

46. Pull-Up

Starting Position • Standing under the pull-up bar (or the alternative device you have selected or fabricated), jump up and grasp the bar with *the palms of the hands facing away from you*. Do *not* grasp the bar with the palms facing toward you. Dangle from the bar with the arms relaxed and fully extended. (Be sure the bar is high enough so you can do this.)

Execution • ONE   Lift the body slowly and smoothly until you can touch the top of the bar with the bottom of the chin (or, better yet, with the upper part of the throat). Keep the legs together but relaxed beneath you. Pause.

TWO   Recover to the starting position by easing the body slowly downward. Do not simply drop, and do not rest the toes or feet on the ground, if the ground is reachable. Come to a complete stop before beginning the next cycle.

Comments • As are most push-ups, most pull-ups are done incorrectly and therefore ineffectively. The single most common error is grasping the bar with the palms facing toward you instead of away from you. Other errors include not lifting the chin over the bar; allowing the toes to touch the ground on the TWO counts; and not pausing at the end of each count. You will find that most people who boast of doing fifteen or twenty pull-ups do them incorrectly. (Try both ways, to experience the difference for yourself.)

Do not begin the first ONE count until you are dangling from the bar as a dead weight, with the arms fully extended.

Once you have tried a few Pull-Ups, *performed correctly,* you'll see why this exercise is truly outstanding as an arm and chest strengthener.

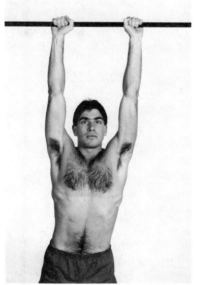

(Pull-Up) Starting and finishing position

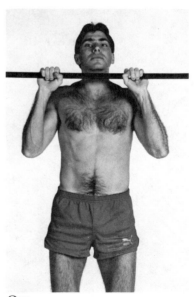

One

Table 2:
Schedule for the Calisthenics Program

	Week 1					Week 2				
Exercise Session:	1	2	3	4	5	6	7	8	9	10
1. Full Jumping Jack	20	25	25	30	30	20	20	20	20	20
2. Half Jumping Jack	20	20	20	20	20	20	20	20	20	20
3. Side Twister Stretcher	—	—	—	—	10	15	14	15	15	15
4. Trunk Rotation	10	12	12	12	12	—	12	—	—	—
5. Trunk Bending Fore and Aft	10	12	12	12	16	14	—	12	—	15
6. Trunk Twister	10	12	12	14	15	10	—	—	10	10
7. Windmill, Four-Count	—	—	—	—	10	8	—	—	—	8
8. Windmill, Two-Count	—	—	10	—	10	16	—	15	—	17
9. Trunk Side Stretcher	10	12	12	14	15	—	—	—	8	—
10. Rocking Chair	—	—	—	—	—	—	—	12	12	—
11. Regulation Sit-Up	—	25	15	—	—	18	—	20	—	19
12. Hand-and-Toe Sit-Up	10	—	—	15	16	—	14	—	15	—
13. Cherry Picker	10	12	14	15	—	—	12	12	12	12
14. Back Flutter Kick	100	100	100	100	100	100	—	100	100	100
15. Stomach Flutter Kick	—	—	—	75	80	—	60	—	60	60
16. Sitting Flutter Kick	50	55	—	75	80	30	40	40	40	—
17. Back Roller	—	6	8	8	10	—	—	—	—	—
18. Stomach Stretcher	4	5	6	7	8	8	8	8	8	9
19. Sitting Knee Bend	—	—	—	—	10	—	10	—	—	—
20. Leg Lever	—	—	—	—	—	—	—	—	—	—
21. Leg Thrust	—	—	—	—	—	—	14	15	15	16
22. Legs Flexing, Shoulders Secured	—	—	—	6	6	8	8	6	8	—
23. Back Flexing, Legs Secured	—	—	—	6	6	8	8	6	8	—
24. Side Flexing, Legs Secured	—	—	—	6	6	8	8	6	6	—
25. Sitting Back Bends	10	10	—	—	10	10	—	10	—	—
26. Side Snapper	—	—	—	—	—	—	—	—	—	—
27. Deep Knee Bender, Four-Count	15	—	—	—	18	—	20	—	—	—
28. Deep Knee Bender, Two-Count	—	20	18	—	20	20	20	20	—	20
29. Squat Jump	—	—	—	—	—	10	10	10	10	10
30. Leg Stretcher	10	8	8	10	8	10	8	10	10	10
31. Thigh Stretcher	—	6	7	10	10	10	8	10	10	10
32. Groin Stretcher, Four-Count	—	—	—	—	—	6	—	—	—	—
33. Groin Stretcher, Two-Count	—	—	—	—	—	8	—	—	—	—
34. Calf Stretcher	—	—	10	—	—	—	8	—	10	—
35. One-Legged Sit-Up	—	—	—	10	—	—	—	—	—	—
36. Bend and Reach	—	—	—	10	—	—	—	—	—	—
37. Squat Stretch	—	—	—	10	—	—	—	—	—	10
38. Good Morning Darling	10	—	16	—	15	20	20	15	—	21
39. Spread Eagle	—	—	—	—	—	—	—	—	—	—
40. Deep Breather	—	—	—	—	—	4	—	—	—	6
41. Eight-Count Body Builder	10	10	10	10	12	8	—	10	8	9
42. Neck Rotation	—	—	—	—	—	9	—	—	—	8
43. One-Legged Push-Up	—	—	—	—	—	—	24	—	26	—
44. Press Press Fling	10	10	10	10	10	8	10	10	10	10
45. Up Back and Over	10	10	10	10	10	8	10	10	10	10
46. Pull-Up	2	2	3	3	3	3	3	3	3	3

Table 2 (cont'd)

Week 3					Week 4					Week 5					Week 6				
11	12	13	14	15	16	17	18	19	20	21	22	23	24	25	26	27	28	29	30
25	30	35	35	40	45	22	30	35	40	40	40	35	40	30	50	35	40	50	50
20	20	—	20	—	—	20	20	—	—	—	20	20	—	20	—	20	20	—	—
15	—	—	16	—	14	16	16	16	—	16	16	—	16	16	—	18	—	18	—
12	12	14	—	14	15	16	—	16	16	—	18	18	—	18	20	—	—	20	20
—	—	—	—	16	—	—	—	15	16	16	—	16	16	—	—	16	16	18	18
—	—	10	—	12	—	10	10	—	16	10	—	12	12	—	13	14	15	—	—
—	—	—	—	—	12	—	—	8	8	10	—	10	10	—	10	—	—	—	20
—	—	—	—	—	18	—	—	24	24	24	—	—	25	25	—	26	26	27	27
8	8	8	—	10	14	8	8	—	16	—	10	10	10	10	—	—	—	10	10
12	12	12	12	10	—	14	—	—	—	—	18	18	—	—	19	—	—	—	—
—	—	—	20	—	20	—	—	27	—	28	—	29	—	30	—	32	33	34	—
15	15	16	—	18	—	18	19	—	20	—	22	—	23	—	24	—	—	—	25
—	—	—	—	—	12	—	—	12	12	12	—	—	12	—	—	12	14	—	—
120	120	125	130	135	140	130	—	140	150	150	175	175	—	175	175	200	200	200	215
—	—	—	—	85	—	—	60	—	100	—	—	—	65	—	—	—	—	—	75
—	—	—	—	85	90	—	40	40	60	—	—	—	45	—	45	—	—	—	—
8	8	8	8	8	10	8	8	—	—	—	10	—	10	—	10	—	—	—	—
10	11	12	13	14	15	15	16	—	—	—	18	—	19	20	—	22	23	—	24
—	—	—	—	—	—	—	—	—	—	—	15	—	—	16	—	—	—	—	—
—	—	—	—	—	—	—	—	10	10	10	—	—	10	—	—	10	12	12	12
16	—	16	16	—	18	20	21	22	25	25	28	—	29	—	30	—	—	—	—
8	8	8	8	—	8	8	8	—	10	10	—	10	—	10	—	10	10	10	10
8	8	8	8	—	8	8	8	—	10	10	—	10	—	10	—	10	10	10	10
6	6	6	6	—	8	6	6	—	6	6	—	6	—	8	—	8	8	8	8
10	10	10	—	10	—	—	10	10	10	10	—	10	10	10	10	12	12	12	12
—	—	—	—	—	—	—	—	—	—	—	8	—	—	8	—	8	8	10	10
—	20	—	15	20	20	—	—	—	—	—	12	—	12	—	—	—	—	—	—
20	—	20	20	—	—	20	20	—	22	22	22	—	22	20	—	22	22	—	—
10	11	12	12	—	15	16	16	16	16	17	—	18	—	19	20	—	—	22	22
10	10	10	10	10	10	10	10	10	10	10	10	—	10	10	10	10	12	12	12
10	—	10	10	10	10	10	10	10	10	10	10	—	10	10	10	10	12	12	12
—	—	—	—	—	8	—	—	6	6	—	7	—	8	—	10	—	—	—	—
—	—	—	—	—	6	—	—	8	8	—	8	—	10	—	—	10	10	—	—
—	—	—	10	—	—	—	—	—	—	8	—	—	—	—	8	—	—	—	—
—	—	—	—	—	—	—	—	—	—	—	4	—	4	—	5	—	6	6	6
—	—	—	—	—	—	—	—	—	—	—	8	—	—	—	—	8	8	8	8
—	—	—	—	—	—	10	—	—	—	8	—	—	—	—	—	—	—	—	6
15	15	20	20	20	20	—	30	20	20	20	15	—	35	20	25	—	15	15	20
—	—	—	—	10	—	—	—	—	—	—	—	10	—	—	10	—	—	—	—
4	4	6	—	—	—	—	6	—	—	6	4	6	6	6	—	6	6	6	6
9	9	10	—	14	12	10	10	—	—	—	12	—	12	—	12	—	—	—	12
—	—	—	—	—	—	—	—	10	—	10	—	10	—	—	—	10	—	10	—
—	—	—	30	—	—	—	—	30	30	32	—	34	—	35	—	36	36	37	37
10	10	10	10	10	10	8	10	8	8	8	10	10	10	12	8	10	10	10	10
10	10	10	10	10	10	8	10	—	—	8	10	10	10	8	8	10	10	—	—
4	4	4	4	4	4	4	4	4	4	5	5	5	5	5	5	5	5	5	5

Table 2 (cont'd)

Exercise Session:	31	32	33	34	35	36	37	38	39	40
			Week 7					Week 8		
1. Full Jumping Jack	45	45	45	45	50	50	75	75	40	40
2. Half Jumping Jack	—	20	20	20	20	20	—	—	20	12
3. Side Twister Stretcher	—	18	18	18	18	—	—	16	18	—
4. Trunk Rotation	20	—	16	—	16	18	20	18	—	18
5. Trunk Bending Fore and Aft	—	18	18	18	16	18	—	10	18	18
6. Trunk Twister	16	10	—	10	—	—	—	—	14	14
7. Windmill, Four-Count	—	—	—	—	—	—	10	—	12	14
8. Windmill, Two-Count	28	—	—	—	—	—	30	30	—	14
9. Trunk Side Stretcher	10	10	12	10	12	12	10	—	—	—
10. Rocking Chair	—	22	22	23	24	—	—	—	25	—
11. Regulation Sit-Up	35	—	—	—	—	—	—	40	—	—
12. Hand-and-Toe Sit-Up	—	27	28	28	28	29	29	—	29	30
13. Cherry Picker	—	12	14	13	13	15	12	12	12	12
14. Back Flutter Kick	225	—	250	255	255	260	275	—	300	300
15. Stomach Flutter Kick	75	100	110	100	110	100	100	100	—	—
16. Sitting Flutter Kick	—	60	70	70	75	80	—	60	—	—
17. Back Roller	—	10	10	10	10	10	10	—	12	12
18. Stomach Stretcher	25	—	—	—	—	26	—	—	29	30
19. Sitting Knee Bend	—	18	18	18	18	18	20	—	—	—
20. Leg Lever	12	—	—	—	—	—	—	12	—	—
21. Leg Thrust	—	33	33	33	33	33	37	—	—	—
22. Legs Flexing, Shoulders Secured	12	—	—	—	—	—	—	—	12	12
23. Back Flexing, Legs Secured	12	—	—	—	—	—	—	—	12	12
24. Side Flexing, Legs Secured	8	—	—	—	—	—	—	—	8	8
25. Sitting Back Bends	10	12	12	12	12	12	12	10	10	10
26. Side Snapper	—	12	12	12	12	12	—	10	—	10
27. Deep Knee Bender, Four-Count	—	—	—	—	—	20	25	20	—	—
28. Deep Knee Bender, Two-Count	—	—	—	—	—	—	25	20	—	—
29. Squat Jump	23	24	24	24	25	24	25	—	25	26
30. Leg Stretcher	12	12	—	12	12	12	12	10	12	12
31. Thigh Stretcher	10	12	—	12	12	—	12	10	10	10
32. Groin Stretcher, Four-Count	—	10	—	10	—	—	8	—	—	—
33. Groin Stretcher, Two-Count	—	—	10	—	10	—	12	—	—	—
34. Calf Stretcher	—	10	10	10	10	12	10	—	—	—
35. One-Legged Sit-Up	—	6	6	6	6	—	—	—	6	8
36. Bend and Reach	8	—	—	8	—	—	—	10	12	12
37. Squat Stretch	—	—	—	—	—	—	10	—	—	—
38. Good Morning Darling	25	30	30	31	31	32	—	—	10	10
39. Spread Eagle	12	—	—	—	—	—	—	18	—	—
40. Deep Breather	6	—	—	—	—	—	—	—	6	6
41. Eight-Count Body Builder	—	14	15	14	15	17	—	16	—	—
42. Neck Rotation	10	—	—	—	—	—	10	10	—	—
43. One-Legged Push-Up	38	—	—	—	—	—	42	—	44	44
44. Press Press Fling	10	12	12	12	12	12	10	10	—	—
45. Up Back and Over	8	—	—	—	—	12	—	10	—	—
46. Pull-Up	6	6	6	6	6	6	6	6	6	6

Table 2 (cont'd)

Week 9					Week 10					Week 11					Week 12				
41	42	43	44	45	46	47	48	49	50	51	52	53	54	55	56	57	58	59	60
40	50	75	50	50	50	50	50	50	50	50	50	50	50	50	50	50	50	50	50
12	20	20	—	20	20	20	20	20	20	20	20	—	20	20	—	20	20	20	20
—	20	—	20	—	20	—	20	20	—	—	20	—	20	20	—	—	20	20	—
—	—	20	20	15	—	15	—	—	16	16	16	18	20	—	16	16	—	—	16
18	15	14	18	20	20	20	20	20	20	20	—	20	20	20	—	20	20	20	20
16	—	20	20	20	20	20	20	20	20	20	20	20	20	20	20	20	20	20	20
18	—	—	12	—	—	20	—	—	20	22	20	—	—	20	—	20	20	20	20
—	—	40	—	25	—	20	30	30	—	—	20	—	—	20	—	35	26	26	20
16	20	—	12	—	20	20	20	20	20	20	20	20	20	—	20	20	20	20	20
—	25	—	—	—	—	—	20	20	—	—	20	—	—	—	20	—	—	—	—
—	44	—	48	—	50	—	—	—	—	—	—	—	—	—	50	—	—	—	—
31	—	32	—	30	—	32	34	34	—	40	—	42	44	45	—	48	—	—	50
14	15	—	—	—	20	20	—	—	20	20	20	20	20	20	20	20	—	—	10
300	—	—	325	330	—	335	340	340	345	350	—	360	365	370	—	350	375	375	400
115	—	140	—	—	100	100	—	—	110	—	—	120	125	—	—	130	135	135	—
100	—	80	—	—	150	150	150	155	150	—	170	175	180	125	125	—	—	—	—
—	—	12	—	—	10	10	—	—	—	12	—	—	—	—	—	10	—	—	10
31	—	—	31	32	33	—	35	35	—	—	38	40	41	35	35	—	—	—	50
—	20	23	—	—	20	20	—	—	22	20	—	—	—	—	—	—	—	—	—
—	15	—	15	—	20	—	—	—	—	—	—	—	—	20	20	—	—	—	—
—	40	39	—	20	—	20	—	—	30	—	30	—	—	—	—	—	35	35	—
12	—	10	10	10	—	12	—	—	12	12	—	12	12	12	12	12	—	—	—
12	—	10	10	10	—	12	—	—	12	12	—	12	12	12	12	12	—	—	—
8	—	10	10	—	—	12	—	—	12	12	—	12	12	12	12	12	—	—	—
12	10	10	12	12	12	12	12	12	12	12	12	12	12	—	12	—	—	12	12
—	—	12	—	—	—	—	—	—	—	—	—	—	—	—	—	—	—	—	—
—	30	—	—	30	30	—	30	30	25	30	30	—	—	30	—	30	30	30	—
—	—	—	30	—	—	30	—	—	25	—	35	—	—	40	—	40	35	35	—
26	—	25	—	—	—	—	—	—	—	—	—	—	—	—	—	—	—	—	—
12	10	12	12	12	12	12	12	12	12	12	12	12	12	10	12	12	12	12	12
12	10	10	12	12	12	12	12	12	12	12	12	12	12	12	12	15	12	12	12
10	—	—	10	—	10	—	12	12	—	—	14	—	14	—	—	—	16	16	16
10	—	—	—	12	10	—	12	12	—	—	14	—	14	—	—	—	16	16	16
—	—	10	10	—	—	—	12	12	—	—	—	—	—	—	—	15	20	20	—
—	—	—	8	—	—	10	12	12	—	—	12	—	12	—	—	—	—	—	—
15	—	—	10	—	—	10	—	—	—	—	—	12	—	—	—	—	—	—	—
—	8	8	—	—	—	—	—	—	—	—	—	—	—	—	—	—	—	8	—
15	50	50	30	30	30	—	—	—	30	—	—	—	—	—	32	—	—	—	—
—	—	—	12	12	—	—	20	20	—	—	—	—	—	—	—	—	—	—	—
—	—	6	—	6	—	6	—	6	—	6	—	6	—	6	—	6	—	6	—
18	—	18	—	—	20	22	22	22	22	22	—	22	—	24	—	24	—	24	25
—	10	—	10	—	—	—	—	—	—	—	—	—	—	—	—	—	—	—	—
—	45	—	40	46	—	—	—	—	—	—	50	—	50	—	52	—	54	54	—
12	—	8	—	10	10	10	12	12	12	12	12	12	12	12	12	12	12	12	12
12	8	—	—	10	10	10	12	12	12	12	12	12	12	12	12	12	12	12	12
7	7	7	7	7	7	7	7	7	7	8	8	8	8	8	8	8	9	9	10

The Running Program

No other single, readily accessible activity is more beneficial to the physical conditioning of the human body than regular running. Only swimming is generally regarded as being a better conditioner, but few people have access to swimming on a regular basis.

In essence, running does it all. It builds up the strength and stamina of the body's primary means of locomotion (and survival); it builds up the capacity of the respiratory and circulatory systems to sustain intense as well as protracted durations of physical effort; it heightens the threshold of pain; and it provides euphoric feelings of accomplishment that build self-confidence and self-esteem. And no less importantly, running serves to purge the mind and body of physical and psychological tension—or, as a colleague of mine would say of running, "It blows out the pipes."

Running is considered so important to the conditioning of the U.S. Navy frogmen and SEALs that, not only is the trainee required to complete the same amount of running required by the twelve-week Running Program presented in this book (running up to eight miles a day), he (or she) is also required to run or double-time every place he goes during the entire time he is in the frogman/SEAL training program. In other words, the trainee never walks from the moment he enters the training program to the moment he officially completes it. (The habit is hard to break: sixteen years after completing the training program, I'm still running up to fourteen miles a day.)

The Conditioning Hike

With tongue firmly in cheek, the Navy refers to its training runs for frogman and SEAL trainees as "conditioning hikes." These conditioning hikes are more than runs, however, and certainly more than walks, so the term is probably more appropriate than the apparent irony of the term would suggest.

The conditioning hike alternates between periods of running and periods of walking (double-timing), and most of the running periods terminate with a brief period of sprinting. Typically, a hike is conducted on a varying topography of ocean-beach sand; from soft to hard-packed, from steeply duned to well submerged in the surf. And typically it is run in a pair of heavy boots. The variations in tempo and topography, and the heavy boots, are designed to add further demands that must be met with additional effort (mental as well as physical). The trainee thereby gains more conditioning benefit to the mile.

You will not be required to take up residence near the ocean so that you can run in beach sand. However, it is strongly recommended that you choose running routes that provide a varied topography. In other words, run up all the hills you can find. It is also recommended that you wear heavy boots instead of featherweight running shoes.

Frogman and SEAL trainees are not expected to run eight miles on their first outing; so relax—you aren't either. In fact, you are only required to run for a total of fifteen minutes on the first outing, covering a distance of about two miles. And this distance is broken up by several intervals of fast walking. Thereafter the running requirements gradually progress until, in the fourth week, they reach a maximum of about eight miles (sixty minutes).

Techniques and Suggestions

The following techniques and suggestions are used by most Navy frogman and SEAL trainees to help "get them through" the running program, not only successfully but as painlessly as possible. You should find them equally as useful.

- While running, strive to keep all the muscles of your body as relaxed as possible—even those in your legs. Do this by making a habit of being consciously aware of the status of your muscles, especially those that are prone to become tense when the body is under stress (those in the lower back, in the upper arms, and in the shoulders and neck). If you do not do this, you may develop sore muscles much earlier than you would normally (and in places you might not expect to); you might even suffer cramps.
- Wearing ankle weights or heavy boots (jump or combat boots) is strongly recommended, because of the increased weight they provide; however, wearing boots can increase the incidence of friction blisters on the feet. To limit the possibility of developing blisters from boots made of leather, thoroughly soak your boots in warm water and walk them dry (wear them all day).

  If your boots should subsequently become wet—from rain, for example—do not dry them in direct sunlight, or in any other direct-heat source, as this may cause the leather to stiffen and shrink, thereby increasing the likelihood of blistering.

  If your feet tend to slip around in your boots, wear an extra pair of socks (preferably cotton). If you wear ankle weights, be sure to protect your legs from chafing.
- Running is never comfortable, and is often quite the

contrary. Your brain is going to recognize this fact very early on, and is probably going to react by trying to convince you to quit, at least for the day, by all manner of ploys; but mainly, I suspect, by singing you such seductive songs as "There's Always Tomorrow" and "Wouldn't It Feel *Good* to Walk the Rest of the Way" and "Nobody's Lookin' So It's Okay to Walk." There's no way to silence these seductions, but you can choose not to hear them. In other words, you can choose to distract yourself in some way. Daydream, for example, or fantasize running the Boston Marathon, or problem-solve, or plan your day, or remember a fond moment, or simply watch the scenery. You might also find it helpful to change your route frequently, as a way of providing yourself with fresh distractions. One thing *not* to do, however, is to keep looking up the road in front of you to note how little you seem to have progressed in what seems to have been the last century. (When I'm feeling beleaguered, I find it best to keep my eyes on the road, with my thoughts turned inward.)

- To lessen the possibility of your legs becoming stiff and sore after a run, especially after a demanding one, keep your legs as active as possible. First, do the recommended stretching exercises, then walk as much as you can. If you cannot keep your legs "actively" active ("proactive" if you're into jargon), then choose standing over sitting. The intent is to keep the blood circulating in your legs as vigorously as possible.

- Do not consume alcoholic beverages immediately before or after a run. Alcohol is a diuretic and will tend to dehydrate you. Also avoid coffee, citrus, and bananas, which may tend to give you heartburn while you are running. To simplify things, drink water—and only water—before, during, and after a run. And drink plenty of it.

- Try not to eat or drink anything except water for at least three hours before running. If you have to eat immediately before exercising or running, eat lightly, and avoid like the plague such things as meats, dairy products, and rich or spicy foods (pizza, pastries, and the like). If you're trying to lose weight, here's a tip: plan your workout sessions to immediately precede a major meal; then eat as soon after each session as you can. You should find yourself eating much less than normally. (Don't wait too long, though, as your appetite will tend to increase with the length of time lapsed after the completion of a session.)
- If you can, begin the scheduled run within five to ten minutes of completing the day's quota of calisthenics. If you cannot do this, be sure to do some stretching exercises (see the Stretching Program) before you run.
- If the weather is warm, wear a sweatband to keep perspiration from stinging your eyes.
- If the weather is cold, put on two or three thin layers of clothing rather than one heavy layer. Then you can peel off layers as you warm up. Wear a hat and gloves (or mittens); and wear something that has a pouch or deep pockets, to put things in, including your hat or gloves, as you need to take them off. If you wish to invest in clothing that is specially made for cold-weather running, Moss Brown and Company is an excellent source (catalog: 5210 Eisenhower Avenue, Alexandria, Va. 22304).
- Also for cool or cold weather, put newspaper or Vaseline over your nipples (if male); otherwise, they may stiffen from the cool air and chafe against your sweaty clothing. This can be *very* uncomfortable. If female, wear a quality running bra.
- If male, you may find running briefs (available at any sporting goods store) more comfortable than the tra-

ditional athletic supporter. If female, wear a running bra rather than a regular bra, for better support.

The Program and Schedule

The Running Program consists of daily schedules of alternate running and rapid walking (double-timing). As the program progresses, the periods of running become longer and the periods of walking become shorter. The running periods include brief intervals of sprinting. A complete (detachable) schedule for the Running Program is provided at the end of this section (Table 3); week-by-week schedules are provided in the section entitled Schedules.

Because the various intervals of running, sprinting, and walking need to be timed (this is a time-based program, not a distance-based program), you should wear a watch during each hike, preferably one with a stop-watch capability. Plastic watches are more appropriate than metal watches, because plastic watches are lighter, do not flop around on the wrist, and do not irritate or discolor the skin.

During the scheduled running intervals, you should maintain a steady pace of from 180 to 200 paces per minute, which is equivalent to about eight miles per hour. During the walking intervals, you should double-time. Normal walking speed is about three miles per hour; double-time speed is five to six miles per hour.

For Hikes 1–6, double your speed to 360 paces per minute (fourteen miles per hour) during the final *thirty seconds* of each running interval; for Hikes 7–60, run at the very fastest rate you can (pretend you're being chased by a rabid Doberman pinscher) during the last *sixty seconds* of each running interval.

Table 3:
Schedule for the Running Program
(in minutes)

Hike#:	Week 1					Week 2					Week 3					Week 4					Weeks 5–12 21–60
	1	2	3	4	5	6	7	8	9	10	11	12	13	14	15	16	17	18	19	20	
Run	3	4	4	4	5	5	6	6	6	7	7	8	8	9	9	10	11	15	20	25	25
Walk	6	6	6	6	6	6	6	6	6	4	4	3	3	2	2	1	1	1	1	5	5
Run	3	4	4	4	5	5	6	6	6	7	7	8	8	9	9	10	11	30	10	20	20
Walk	6	6	6	6	6	6	6	6	6	4	4	3	3	2	2	1	1	1	1	10	10
Run	3	4	4	4	5	5	6	6	6	7	7	8	8	9	9	10	11	15	30	—	—
Walk	6	6	6	6	6	6	6	6	6	4	4	3	3	2	2	1	1	10	10	—	—
Run	3	4	4	4	5	5	6	6	6	7	7	8	8	9	9	10	11	—	—	—	—
Walk	6	6	6	6	6	6	6	6	6	4	4	3	3	2	2	1	1	—	—	—	—
Run	3	4	4	4	5	5	6	6	6	7	7	8	8	9	9	10	10	—	—	—	—
Walk	10	10	10	10	10	10	10	10	10	10	10	10	10	10	10	10	10	—	—	—	—
Total Run Time	15	20	20	20	25	25	30	30	30	35	35	40	40	45	45	50	55	60	60	45	45
Total Walk Time	34	34	34	34	34	34	34	34	34	26	26	22	22	18	18	14	14	12	12	15	15

Schedules

Week 0

Use this week to prepare yourself, mentally, physically, and logistically.

- Read this book through *completely*—twice if possible.
- Try each exercise, paying particular attention to learning the proper form.
- Practice the more difficult exercises, but without worrying about achieving mastery at this time.
- Gather all the clothing and equipment you will need (shoes or boots, plastic running watch, sweatband, etc.).
- Provide yourself access to a pull-up bar.
- Tell somebody what you are about to do, to help pressure yourself into actually doing it.
- Consciously commit yourself to seeing the program through to the very end of the twelfth week.
- Plan to give yourself a reward at the end of each week (your choice), and a *special* reward at the end of the overall program.
- Have someone take a "before" picture of you showing as much skin as you're willing to expose. (Don't miss out on this before-and-after opportunity, especially if you're entering this program as a nonathlete.)
- Finally, take your at-rest pulse rate (at the same time of day you will be exercising) and record it in the Per-

sonal Record Chart provided in this book (page 166). (The normal range for nonathletes is seventy to seventy-five beats per minute.) You may also wish to record your weight, waist or hip size, biceps, and thighs.

Week 1:
Calisthenics Schedule

	Repetitions per Session				
Exercise Session#:	1	2	3	4	5
1. Full Jumping Jack	20	25	25	30	30
2. Half Jumping Jack	20	20	20	20	20
3. Side Twister Stretcher	—	—	—	—	10
4. Trunk Rotation	10	12	12	12	12
5. Trunk Bending Fore and Aft	10	12	12	12	16
6. Trunk Twister	10	12	12	14	15
7. Windmill, Four-Count	—	—	—	—	10
8. Windmill, Two-Count	—	—	10	—	10
9. Trunk Side Stretcher	10	12	12	14	15
11. Regulation Sit-Up	—	25	15	—	—
12. Hand-and-Toe Sit-Up	10	—	—	15	16
13. Cherry Picker	10	12	14	15	—
14. Back Flutter Kick	100	100	100	100	100
15. Stomach Flutter Kick	—	—	—	75	80
16. Sitting Flutter Kick	50	55	—	75	80
17. Back Roller	—	6	8	8	10
18. Stomach Stretcher	4	5	6	7	8
19. Sitting Knee Bend	—	—	—	—	10
22. Legs Flexing, Shoulders Secured	—	—	—	6	6
23. Back Flexing, Legs Secured	—	—	—	6	6
24. Side Flexing, Legs Secured	—	—	—	6	6
25. Sitting Back Bends	10	10	—	—	10
27. Deep Knee Bender, Four-Count	15	—	—	—	18
28. Deep Knee Bender, Two-Count	—	20	18	—	20
30. Leg Stretcher	10	8	8	10	8
31. Thigh Stretcher	—	6	7	10	10
34. Calf Stretcher	—	—	10	—	—

Exercise Session#:	Repetitions per Session				
	1	2	3	4	5
36. Bend and Reach	—	—	—	10	—
37. Squat Stretch	—	—	—	10	—
38. Good Morning Darling	10	—	16	—	15
41. Eight-Count Body Builder	10	10	10	10	12
44. Press Press Fling	10	10	10	10	10
45. Up Back and Over	10	10	10	10	10
46. Pull-Up	2	2	3	3	3

Week 1:
Running Schedule

Hike#:	Minutes per Hike				
	1	2	3	4	5
Run/Sprint	3	4	4	4	5
Walk	6	6	6	6	6
Run/Sprint	3	4	4	4	5
Walk	6	6	6	6	6
Run/Sprint	3	4	4	4	5
Walk	6	6	6	6	6
Run/Sprint	3	4	4	4	5
Walk	6	6	6	6	6
Run/Sprint	3	4	4	4	5
Walk	10	10	10	10	10
Total Run Time	15	20	20	20	25
Total Walk Time	34	34	34	34	34

Comments

- Exercises 22, 23, and 24, introduced in Session 4, are best performed with a partner, especially when you are first learning them. Therefore, you may wish to have someone available to help you with these.
- Go slowly this week, concentrating on proper form and correct execution. Refer back to the descriptions and illustrations as necessary.
- Don't forget to include the Stretching Program in your workouts if at all possible.

- Choose a space to exercise in that will allow you to perform the Full Jumping Jack (arms extended over the head) and the Squat Stretch (two-foot jump into the air).
- And don't forget your reward at the end of the week!

Week 2:
Calisthenics Schedule

		Repetitions per Session			
Exercise Session#:	6	7	8	9	10
1. Full Jumping Jack	20	20	20	20	20
2. Half Jumping Jack	20	20	20	20	20
3. Side Twister Stretcher	15	14	15	15	15
4. Trunk Rotation	—	12	—	—	—
5. Trunk Bending Fore and Aft	14	—	12	—	15
6. Trunk Twister	10	—	—	10	10
7. Windmill, Four-Count	8	—	—	—	8
8. Windmill, Two-Count	16	—	15	—	17
9. Trunk Side Stretcher	—	—	—	8	—
10. Rocking Chair	—	—	12	12	—
11. Regulation Sit-Up	18	—	20	—	19
12. Hand-and-Toe Sit-Up	—	14	—	15	—
13. Cherry Picker	—	12	12	12	12
14. Back Flutter Kick	100	—	100	100	100
15. Stomach Flutter Kick	—	60	—	60	60
16. Sitting Flutter Kick	30	40	40	40	—
18. Stomach Stretcher	8	8	8	8	9
19. Sitting Knee Bend	—	10	—	—	—
21. Leg Thrust	—	14	15	15	16
22. Legs Flexing, Shoulders Secured	8	8	6	8	—
23. Back Flexing, Legs Secured	8	8	6	8	—
24. Side Flexing, Legs Secured	8	8	6	6	—
25. Sitting Back Bends	10	—	10	—	—
27. Deep Knee Bender, Four-Count	—	20	—	—	—
28. Deep Knee Bender, Two-Count	20	20	20	—	20

	Repetitions per Session				
Exercise Session#:	6	7	8	9	10
29. Squat Jump	10	10	10	10	10
30. Leg Stretcher	10	8	10	10	10
31. Thigh Stretcher	10	8	10	10	10
32. Groin Stretcher, Four-Count	6	—	—	—	—
33. Groin Stretcher, Two-Count	8	—	—	—	—
34. Calf Stretcher	—	8	—	10	—
37. Squat Stretch	—	—	—	—	10
38. Good Morning Darling	20	20	15	—	21
40. Deep Breather	4	—	—	—	6
41. Eight-Count Body Builder	8	—	10	8	9
42. Neck Rotation	9	—	—	—	8
43. One-Legged Push-Up	—	24	—	26	—
44. Press Press Fling	8	10	10	10	10
45. Up Back and Over	8	10	10	10	10
46. Pull-Up	3	3	3	3	3

Boldface indicates first appearance of this exercise in the schedules.

Week 2:
Running Schedule

	Minutes per Hike				
Hike#:	6	7	8	9	10
Run/Sprint	5	6	6	6	7
Walk	6	6	6	6	4
Run/Sprint	5	6	6	6	7
Walk	6	6	6	6	4
Run/Sprint	5	6	6	6	7
Walk	6	6	6	6	4
Run/Sprint	5	6	6	6	7
Walk	6	6	6	6	4
Run/Sprint	5	6	6	6	7
Walk	10	10	10	10	10
Total Run Time	25	30	30	30	35
Total Walk Time	34	34	34	34	26

Comments

- Several new exercises this week: the Rocking Chair; the Leg Thrust; the Squat Jump; the Groin Stretcher, Four-Count; the Groin Stretcher, Two-Count; the Deep Breather; the Neck Rotation; and the One-Legged Push-Up. You may wish to practice these exercises a few times before you have to do them in earnest. This is especially true of the Squat Jump and the Groin Stretchers—which are *not* easy exercises.
- Be patient with these new exercises. Mastery should be a goal, not an immediate expectation.
- Thorough before-workout stretching *and* after-workout stretching are highly recommended this week (and every other week!).
- Note that at the end of this week you will be running a full twenty minutes more a day than you ran the first day of the program.

Week 3: Calisthenics Schedule

	Repetitions per Session				
Exercise Session#:	11	12	13	14	15
1. Full Jumping Jack	25	30	35	35	40
2. Half Jumping Jack	20	20	—	20	—
3. Side Twister Stretcher	15	—	—	16	—
4. Trunk Rotation	12	12	14	—	14
5. Trunk Bending Fore and Aft	—	—	—	—	16
6. Trunk Twister	—	—	10	—	12
9. Trunk Side Stretcher	8	8	8	—	10
10. Rocking Chair	12	12	12	12	10
11. Regulation Sit-Up	—	—	—	20	—
12. Hand-and-Toe Sit-Up	15	15	16	—	18
14. Back Flutter Kick	120	120	125	130	135
15. Stomach Flutter Kick	—	—	—	—	85
16. Sitting Flutter Kick	—	—	—	—	85

Exercise Session#:	Repetitions per Session				
	11	12	13	14	15
17. Back Roller	8	8	8	8	8
18. Stomach Stretcher	10	11	12	13	14
21. Leg Thrust	16	—	16	16	—
22. Legs Flexing, Shoulders Secured	8	8	8	8	—
23. Back Flexing, Legs Secured	8	8	8	8	—
24. Side Flexing, Legs Secured	6	6	6	6	—
25. Sitting Back Bends	10	10	10	—	10
27. Deep Knee Bender, Four-Count	—	20	—	15	20
28. Deep Knee Bender, Two-Count	20	—	20	20	—
29. Squat Jump	10	11	12	12	—
30. Leg Stretcher	10	10	10	10	10
31. Thigh Stretcher	10	—	10	10	10
34. Calf Stretcher	—	—	—	10	—
38. Good Morning Darling	15	15	20	20	20
39. Spread Eagle	—	—	—	—	10
40. Deep Breather	4	4	6	—	—
41. Eight-Count Body Builder	9	9	10	—	14
43. One-Legged Push-Up	—	—	—	30	—
44. Press Press Fling	10	10	10	10	10
45. Up Back and Over	10	10	10	10	10
46. Pull-Up	4	4	4	4	4

Week 3:
Running Schedule

Hike#:	Minutes per Hike				
	11	12	13	14	15
Run/Sprint	7	8	8	9	9
Walk	4	3	3	2	2
Run/Sprint	7	8	8	9	9
Walk	4	3	3	2	2
Run/Sprint	7	8	8	9	9
Walk	4	3	3	2	2
Run/Sprint	7	8	8	9	9
Walk	4	3	3	2	2

	Minutes per Hike				
Hike#:	11	12	13	14	15
Run/Sprint	7	8	8	9	9
Walk	10	10	10	10	10
Total Run Time	35	40	40	45	45
Total Walk Time	26	22	22	18	18

Comments

- One new exercise this week: the Spread Eagle. To ensure proper form and execution, review the material on this exercise before performing it.
- To get the most out of those Flutter Kicks (Back, Stomach, and Sitting), you should be wearing boots or ankle weights.
- Keep concentrating on proper form and correct execution—referring back to the descriptions and illustrations as necessary.
- At the end of this week, you will be one-quarter through the program—and you will have *tripled* your running time!

Week 4:
Calisthenics Schedule

	Repetitions per Session				
Exercise Session#:	16	17	18	19	20
1. Full Jumping Jack	45	22	30	35	40
2. Half Jumping Jack	—	20	20	—	—
3. Side Twister Stretcher	14	16	16	16	—
4. Trunk Rotation	15	16	—	16	16
5. Trunk Bending Fore and Aft	—	—	—	15	16
6. Trunk Twister	—	10	10	—	16
7. Windmill, Four-Count	12	—	—	8	8
8. Windmill, Two-Count	18	—	—	24	24
9. Trunk Side Stretcher	14	8	8	—	16

Exercise Session#:	Repetitions per Session				
	16	17	18	19	20
10. Rocking Chair	—	14	—	—	—
11. Regulation Sit-Up	20	—	—	27	—
12. Hand-and-Toe Sit-Up	—	18	19	—	20
13. Cherry Picker	12	—	—	12	12
14. Back Flutter Kick	140	130	—	140	150
15. Stomach Flutter Kick	—	—	60	—	100
16. Sitting Flutter Kick	90	—	40	40	60
17. Back Roller	10	8	8	—	—
18. Stomach Stretcher	15	15	16	—	—
20. Leg Lever	—	—	—	10	10
21. Leg Thrust	18	20	21	22	25
22. Legs Flexing, Shoulders Secured	8	8	8	—	10
23. Back Flexing, Legs Secured	8	8	8	—	10
24. Side Flexing, Legs Secured	8	6	6	—	6
25. Sitting Back Bends	—	—	10	10	10
27. Deep Knee Bender, Four-Count	20	—	—	—	—
28. Deep Knee Bender, Two-Count	—	20	20	—	22
29. Squat Jump	—	15	16	16	16
30. Leg Stretcher	10	10	10	10	10
31. Thigh Stretcher	10	10	10	10	10
32. Groin Stretcher, Four-Count	8	—	—	6	6
33. Groin Stretcher, Two-Count	6	—	—	8	8
37. Squat Stretch	—	10	—	—	—
38. Good Morning Darling	20	—	30	20	20
40. Deep Breather	—	—	6	—	—
41. Eight-Count Body Builder	12	10	10	—	—
42. Neck Rotation	—	—	—	10	—
43. One-Legged Push-Up	—	—	—	30	30
44. Press Press Fling	10	8	10	8	8
45. Up Back and Over	10	8	10	—	—
46. Pull-Up	4	4	4	4	4

Week 4:
Running Schedule

Hike#:	Minutes per Hike				
	16	17	18	19	20
Run/Sprint	10	11	15	20	25
Walk	1	1	1	1	5
Run/Sprint	10	11	30	10	20
Walk	1	1	1	1	10
Run/Sprint	10	11	15	30	—
Walk	1	1	10	10	—
Run/Sprint	10	11	—	—	—
Walk	1	1	—	—	—
Run/Sprint	10	11	—	—	—
Walk	10	10	—	—	—
Total Run Time	50	55	60	60	45
Total Walk Time	14	14	12	12	15

Comments

- One new exercise this week: the Leg Lever. This is another of those exercises that are best performed with a partner. Review the material on this exercise before performing it.
- This is the toughest week of running in the program. Prepare yourself mentally, get plenty of rest, and plan to give yourself an extra reward at the end of this week.

Week 5:
Calisthenics Schedule

Exercise Session#:	21	22	23	24	25
1. Full Jumping Jack	40	40	35	40	30
2. Half Jumping Jack	—	20	20	—	20
3. Side Twister Stretcher	16	16	—	16	16
4. Trunk Rotation	—	18	18	—	18
5. Trunk Bending Fore and Aft	16	—	16	16	—
6. Trunk Twister	10	—	12	12	—
7. Windmill, Four-Count	10	—	10	10	—
8. Windmill, Two-Count	24	—	—	25	25
9. Trunk Side Stretcher	—	10	10	10	10
10. Rocking Chair	—	18	18	—	—
11. Regulation Sit-Up	28	—	29	—	30
12. Hand-and-Toe Sit-Up	—	22	—	23	—
13. Cherry Picker	12	—	—	12	—
14. Back Flutter Kick	150	175	175	—	175
15. Stomach Flutter Kick	—	—	—	65	—
16. Sitting Flutter Kick	—	—	—	45	—
17. Back Roller	—	10	—	10	—
18. Stomach Stretcher	—	18	—	19	20
19. Sitting Knee Bend	—	15	—	—	16
20. Leg Lever	10	—	—	10	—
21. Leg Thrust	25	28	—	29	—
22. Legs Flexing, Shoulders Secured	10	—	10	—	10
23. Back Flexing, Legs Secured	10	—	10	—	10
24. Side Flexing, Legs Secured	6	—	6	—	8
25. Sitting Back Bends	10	—	10	10	10
26. Side Snapper	—	8	—	—	8
27. Deep Knee Bender, Four-Count	—	12	—	12	—
28. Deep Knee Bender, Two-Count	22	22	—	22	20
29. Squat Jump	17	—	18	—	19
30. Leg Stretcher	10	10	10	10	12
31. Thigh Stretcher	10	10	—	10	10
32. Groin Stretcher, Four-Count	—	7	—	8	—

	Repetitions per Session				
Exercise Session#:	21	22	23	24	25
33. Groin Stretcher, Two-Count	—	8	—	10	—
34. Calf Stretcher	8	—	—	—	—
35. One-Legged Sit-Up	—	4	—	4	—
36. Bend and Reach	—	8	—	—	—
37. Squat Stretch	8	—	—	—	—
38. Good Morning Darling	20	15	—	35	20
39. Spread Eagle	—	—	10	—	—
40. Deep Breather	6	4	6	6	6
41. Eight-Count Body Builder	—	12	—	12	—
42. Neck Rotation	10	—	10	—	—
43. One-Legged Push-Up	32	—	34	—	35
44. Press Press Fling	8	10	10	10	12
45. Up Back and Over	8	10	10	10	8
46. Pull-Up	5	5	5	5	5

Week 5:
Running Schedule

	Minutes per Hike				
Hike#:	21	22	23	24	25
Run/Sprint	25	25	25	25	25
Walk	5	5	5	5	5
Run/Sprint	20	20	20	20	20
Walk	10	10	10	10	10
Total Run Time	45	45	45	45	45
Total Walk Time	15	15	15	15	15

Comments

- Two new exercises this week: the Side Snapper and the One-Legged Sit-Up. Review the material on these two exercises before performing them.
- By the end of this week, you will have performed at least twice all forty-six exercises included in the Calisthenics Program.

- Continue to concentrate on mastering proper form and correct execution. To keep yourself reminded of just exactly what the proper form and correct execution are for each exercise, you may wish to review the material on the individual exercises, a few at a time.
- Note that the running time has leveled off to forty-five minutes per session now. From this point on, you may wish to concentrate on increasing your speed—but *gradually*.
- This week begins the final two-thirds of the program—and may be a good time to blaze a new running route, for a change in scenery.

Week 6:
Calisthenics Schedule

	Repetitions per Session				
Exercise Session#:	26	27	28	29	30
1. Full Jumping Jack	50	35	40	50	50
2. Half Jumping Jack	—	20	20	—	—
3. Side Twister Stretcher	—	18	—	18	—
4. Trunk Rotation	20	—	—	20	20
5. Trunk Bending Fore and Aft	—	16	16	18	18
6. Trunk Twister	13	14	15	—	—
7. Windmill, Four-Count	10	—	—	—	20
8. Windmill, Two-Count	—	26	26	27	27
9. Trunk Side Stretcher	10	—	—	10	10
10. Rocking Chair	19	—	—	—	—
11. Regulation Sit-Up	—	32	33	34	—
12. Hand-and-Toe Sit-Up	24	—	—	—	25
13. Cherry Picker	—	12	14	—	—
14. Back Flutter Kick	175	200	200	200	215
15. Stomach Flutter Kick	—	—	—	—	75
16. Sitting Flutter Kick	45	—	—	—	—
17. Back Roller	10	—	—	—	—
18. Stomach Stretcher	—	22	23	—	24
20. Leg Lever	—	10	12	12	12

	Repetitions per Session				
Exercise Session#:	26	27	28	29	30
21. Leg Thrust	30	—	—	—	—
22. Legs Flexing, Shoulders Secured	—	10	10	10	10
23. Back Flexing, Legs Secured	—	10	10	10	10
24. Side Flexing, Legs Secured	—	8	8	8	8
25. Sitting Back Bends	10	12	12	12	12
26. Side Snapper	—	8	8	10	10
28. Deep Knee Bender, Two-Count	—	22	22	—	—
29. Squat Jump	20	—	—	22	22
30. Leg Stretcher	10	12	12	12	12
31. Thigh Stretcher	10	10	12	12	12
32. Groin Stretcher, Four-Count	10	—	—	—	—
33. Groin Stretcher, Two-Count	—	10	10	—	—
34. Calf Stretcher	8	—	—	—	—
35. One-Legged Sit-Up	5	—	6	6	6
36. Bend and Reach	—	8	8	8	8
37. Squat Stretch	—	—	—	—	6
38. Good Morning Darling	25	—	15	15	20
39. Spread Eagle	10	—	—	—	—
40. Deep Breather	—	6	6	6	6
41. Eight-Count Body Builder	12	—	—	—	12
42. Neck Rotation	—	10	—	10	—
43. One-Legged Push-Up	—	36	36	37	37
44. Press Press Fling	8	10	10	10	10
45. Up Back and Over	8	10	10	—	—
46. Pull-Up	5	5	5	5	5

Week 6:
Running Schedule

	Minutes per Hike				
Hike#:	26	27	28	29	30
Run/Sprint	25	25	25	25	25
Walk	5	5	5	5	5
Run/Sprint	20	20	20	20	20
Walk	10	10	10	10	10
Total Run Time	45	45	45	45	45
Total Walk Time	15	15	15	15	15

Comments

- If you haven't been playing music during the calisthenic sessions, you may wish to start doing it—for company, for variety, and for a little added stimulation. Play the kind of music that most stirs you.
- Note that the daily quota for the Back Flutter Kick is continuing to increase steadily—but that your ability to perform it may not be. If you find you're having trouble keeping up, don't worry about it. Just get through the daily quota however you can. If you have to put your legs down for a few moments of rest, do it.
- Are you remembering to count out loud?
- At the end of this week, you will be at the halfway point!

Week 7:
Calisthenics Schedule

	Repetitions per Session				
Exercise Session#:	31	32	33	34	35
1. Full Jumping Jack	45	45	45	45	50
2. Half Jumping Jack	—	20	20	20	20
3. Side Twister Stretcher	—	18	18	18	18
4. Trunk Rotation	20	—	16	—	16
5. Trunk Bending Fore and Aft	—	18	18	18	16
6. Trunk Twister	16	10	—	10	—
8. Windmill, Two-Count	28	—	—	—	—
9. Trunk Side Stretcher	10	10	12	10	12
10. Rocking Chair	—	22	22	23	24
11. Regulation Sit-Up	35	—	—	—	—
12. Hand-and-Toe Sit-Up	—	27	28	28	28
13. Cherry Picker	—	12	14	13	13
14. Back Flutter Kick	225	—	250	255	255
15. Stomach Flutter Kick	75	100	110	100	110
16. Sitting Flutter Kick	—	60	70	70	75
17. Back Roller	—	10	10	10	10

	Repetitions per Session				
Exercise Session#:	31	32	33	34	35
18. Stomach Stretcher	25	—	—	—	—
19. Sitting Knee Bend	—	18	18	18	18
20. Leg Lever	12	—	—	—	—
21. Leg Thrust	—	33	33	33	33
22. Legs Flexing, Shoulders Secured	12	—	—	—	—
23. Back Flexing, Legs Secured	12	—	—	—	—
24. Side Flexing, Legs Secured	8	—	—	—	—
25. Sitting Back Bends	10	12	12	12	12
26. Side Snapper	—	12	12	12	12
29. Squat Jump	23	24	24	24	25
30. Leg Stretcher	12	12	—	12	12
31. Thigh Stretcher	10	12	—	12	12
32. Groin Stretcher, Four-Count	—	10	—	10	—
33. Groin Stretcher, Two-Count	—	—	10	—	10
34. Calf Stretcher	—	10	10	10	10
35. One-Legged Sit-Up	—	6	6	6	6
36. Bend and Reach	8	—	—	8	—
38. Good Morning Darling	25	30	30	31	31
39. Spread Eagle	12	—	—	—	—
40. Deep Breather	6	—	—	—	—
41. Eight-Count Body Builder	—	14	15	14	15
42. Neck Rotation	10	—	—	—	—
43. One-Legged Push-Up	38	—	—	—	—
44. Press Press Fling	10	12	12	12	12
45. Up Back and Over	8	—	—	—	—
46. Pull-Up	6	6	6	6	6

Week 7:
Running Schedule

			Minutes per Hike		
Hike#:	31	32	33	34	35
Run/Sprint	25	25	25	25	25
Walk	5	5	5	5	5
Run/Sprint	20	20	20	20	20
Walk	10	10	10	10	10
Total Run Time	45	45	45	45	45
Total Walk Time	15	15	15	15	15

Comments

- A *lot* of Flutter Kicks (exercises 14, 15, 16) this week. Bear with them. They'll all be worth it in the end.
- Are you continuing to do both before- and after-workout stretching?

Week 8:
Calisthenics Schedule

	Repetitions per Session				
Exercise Session#:	36	37	38	39	40
1. Full Jumping Jack	50	75	75	40	40
2. Half Jumping Jack	20	—	—	20	12
3. Side Twister Stretcher	—	—	16	18	—
4. Trunk Rotation	18	20	18	—	18
5. Trunk Bending Fore and Aft	18	—	10	18	18
6. Trunk Twister	—	—	—	14	14
7. Windmill, Four-Count	—	10	—	12	14
8. Windmill, Two-Count	—	30	30	—	14
9. Trunk Side Stretcher	12	10	—	—	—
10. Rocking Chair	—	—	—	25	—
11. Regulation Sit-Up	—	—	40	—	—
12. Hand-and-Toe Sit-Up	29	29	—	29	30
13. Cherry Picker	15	12	12	12	12

Exercise Session#:	Repetitions per Session				
	36	37	38	39	40
14. Back Flutter Kick	260	275	—	300	300
15. Stomach Flutter Kick	100	100	100	—	—
16. Sitting Flutter Kick	80	—	60	—	—
17. Back Roller	10	10	—	12	12
18. Stomach Stretcher	26	—	—	29	30
19. Sitting Knee Bend	18	20	—	—	—
20. Leg Lever	—	—	12	—	—
21. Leg Thrust	33	37	—	—	—
22. Legs Flexing, Shoulders Secured	—	—	—	12	12
23. Back Flexing, Legs Secured	—	—	—	12	12
24. Side Flexing, Legs Secured	—	—	—	8	8
25. Sitting Back Bends	12	12	10	10	10
26. Side Snapper	12	—	10	—	10
27. Deep Knee Bender, Four-Count	20	25	20	—	—
28. Deep Knee Bender, Two-Count	—	25	20	—	—
29. Squat Jump	24	25	—	25	26
30. Leg Stretcher	12	12	10	12	12
31. Thigh Stretcher	—	12	10	10	10
32. Groin Stretcher, Four-Count	—	8	—	—	—
33. Groin Stretcher, Two-Count	—	12	—	—	—
34. Calf Stretcher	12	10	—	—	—
35. One-Legged Sit-Up	—	—	—	6	8
36. Bend and Reach	—	—	10	12	12
37. Squat Stretch	—	10	—	—	—
38. Good Morning Darling	32	—	—	10	10
39. Spread Eagle	—	—	18	—	—
40. Deep Breather	—	—	—	6	6
41. Eight-Count Body Builder	17	—	16	—	—
42. Neck Rotation	—	10	10	—	—
43. One-Legged Push-Up	—	42	—	44	44
44. Press Press Fling	12	10	10	—	—
45. Up Back and Over	12	—	10	—	—
46. Pull-Up	6	6	6	6	6

Week 8:
Running Schedule

	Minutes per Hike				
Hike#:	36	37	38	39	40
Run/Sprint	25	25	25	25	25
Walk	5	5	5	5	5
Run/Sprint	20	20	20	20	20
Walk	10	10	10	10	10
Total Run Time	45	45	45	45	45
Total Walk Time	15	15	15	15	15

Comments

- At the end of this week, you will be two-thirds through the program!
- You may wish to blaze another new running route this week, for another change in scenery. And if you're playing music during the calisthenic sessions, you may wish to change the records or tapes.

Week 9:
Calisthenics Schedule

	Repetitions per Session				
Exercise Session#:	41	42	43	44	45
1. Full Jumping Jack	40	50	75	50	50
2. Half Jumping Jack	12	20	20	—	20
3. Side Twister Stretcher	—	20	—	20	—
4. Trunk Rotation	—	—	20	20	15
5. Trunk Bending Fore and Aft	18	15	14	18	20
6. Trunk Twister	16	—	20	20	20
7. Windmill, Four-Count	18	—	—	12	—
8. Windmill, Two-Count	—	—	40	—	25
9. Trunk Side Stretcher	16	20	—	12	—
10. Rocking Chair	—	25	—	—	—

Exercise Session#:	Repetitions per Session				
	41	42	43	44	45
11. Regulation Sit-Up	—	44	—	48	—
12. Hand-and-Toe Sit-Up	31	—	32	—	30
13. Cherry Picker	14	15	—	—	—
14. Back Flutter Kick	300	—	—	325	330
15. Stomach Flutter Kick	115	—	140	—	—
16. Sitting Flutter Kick	100	—	80	—	—
17. Back Roller	—	—	12	—	—
18. Stomach Stretcher	31	—	—	31	32
19. Sitting Knee Bend	—	20	23	—	—
20. Leg Lever	—	15	—	15	—
21. Leg Thrust	—	40	39	—	20
22. Legs Flexing, Shoulders Secured	12	—	10	10	10
23. Back Flexing, Legs Secured	12	—	10	10	10
24. Side Flexing, Legs Secured	8	—	10	10	—
25. Sitting Back Bends	12	10	10	12	12
26. Side Snapper	—	—	12	—	—
27. Deep Knee Bender, Four-Count	—	30	—	—	30
28. Deep Knee Bender, Two-Count	—	—	—	30	—
29. Squat Jump	26	—	25	—	—
30. Leg Stretcher	12	10	12	12	12
31. Thigh Stretcher	12	10	10	12	12
32. Groin Stretcher, Four-Count	10	—	—	10	—
33. Groin Stretcher, Two-Count	10	—	—	—	12
34. Calf Stretcher	—	—	10	10	—
35. One-Legged Sit-Up	—	—	—	8	—
36. Bend and Reach	15	—	—	10	—
37. Squat Stretch	—	8	8	—	—
38. Good Morning Darling	15	50	50	30	30
39. Spread Eagle	—	—	—	12	12
40. Deep Breather	—	—	6	—	6
41. Eight-Count Body Builder	18	—	18	—	—
42. Neck Rotation	—	10	—	10	—
43. One-Legged Push-Up	—	45	—	40	46
44. Press Press Fling	12	—	8	—	10
45. Up Back and Over	12	8	—	—	10
46. Pull-Up	7	7	7	7	7

Week 9:
Running Schedule

	Minutes per Hike				
Hike#:	41	42	43	44	45
Run/Sprint	25	25	25	25	25
Walk	5	5	5	5	5
Run/Spring	20	20	20	20	20
Walk	10	10	10	10	10
Total Run Time	45	45	45	45	45
Total Walk Time	15	15	15	15	15

Comments

- At the end of this week, you will be three-quarters through the program!
- Session 41 is National Flutter Kick Day! It may feel like the day you died and went the "wrong way."

Week 10:
Calisthenics Schedule

	Repetitions per Session				
Exercise Session#:	46	47	48	49	50
1. Full Jumping Jack	50	50	50	50	50
2. Half Jumping Jack	20	20	20	20	20
3. Side Twister Stretcher	20	—	20	20	—
4. Trunk Rotation	—	15	—	—	16
5. Trunk Bending Fore and Aft	20	20	20	20	20
6. Trunk Twister	20	20	20	20	20
7. Windmill, Four-Count	—	20	—	—	20
8. Windmill, Two-Count	—	20	30	30	—
9. Trunk Side Stretcher	20	20	20	20	20
10. Rocking Chair	—	—	20	20	—
11. Regulation Sit-Up	50	—	—	—	—

Exercise Session#:	Repetitions per Session				
	46	47	48	49	50
12. Hand-and-Toe Sit-Up	—	32	34	34	—
13. Cherry Picker	20	20	—	—	20
14. Back Flutter Kick	—	335	340	340	345
15. Stomach Flutter Kick	100	100	—	—	110
16. Sitting Flutter Kick	150	150	150	155	150
17. Back Roller	10	10	—	—	—
18. Stomach Stretcher	33	—	35	35	—
19. Sitting Knee Bend	20	20	—	—	22
20. Leg Lever	20	—	—	—	—
21. Leg Thrust	—	20	—	—	30
22. Legs Flexing, Shoulders Secured	—	12	—	—	12
23. Back Flexing, Legs Secured	—	12	—	—	12
24. Side Flexing, Legs Secured	—	12	—	—	12
25. Sitting Back Bends	12	12	12	12	12
27. Deep Knee Bender, Four-Count	30	—	30	30	25
28. Deep Knee Bender, Two-Count	—	30	—	—	25
30. Leg Stretcher	12	12	12	12	12
31. Thigh Stretcher	12	12	12	12	12
32. Groin Stretcher, Four-Count	10	—	12	12	—
33. Groin Stretcher, Two-Count	10	—	12	12	—
34. Calf Stretcher	—	—	12	12	—
35. One-Legged Sit-Up	—	10	12	12	—
36. Bend and Reach	—	10	—	—	—
38. Good Morning Darling	30	—	—	—	30
39. Spread Eagle	—	—	20	20	—
40. Deep Breather	—	6	—	6	—
41. Eight-Count Body Builder	20	22	22	22	22
44. Press Press Fling	10	10	12	12	12
45. Up Back and Over	10	10	12	12	12
46. Pull-Up	7	7	7	7	7

Week 10:
Running Schedule

	Minutes per Hike				
Hike#:	46	47	48	49	50
Run/Sprint	25	25	25	25	25
Walk	5	5	5	5	5
Run/Sprint	20	20	20	20	20
Walk	10	10	10	10	10
Total Run Time	45	45	45	45	45
Total Walk Time	15	15	15	15	15

Comments

- When you see the numbers of Flutter Kicks called for in Sessions 47 and 50, try not to think about them— just get down there and start kicking. And counting. If you have to think about something, think, "Only two more weeks to go!"

Week 11:
Calisthenics Schedule

	Repetitions per Session				
Exercise Session#:	51	52	53	54	55
1. Full Jumping Jack	50	50	50	50	50
2. Half Jumping Jack	20	20	—	20	20
3. Side Twister Stretcher	—	20	—	20	20
4. Trunk Rotation	16	16	18	20	—
5. Trunk Bending Fore and Aft	20	—	20	20	20
6. Trunk Twister	20	20	20	20	20
7. Windmill, Four-Count	22	20	—	—	20
8. Windmill, Two-Count	—	20	—	—	20
9. Trunk Side Stretcher	20	20	20	20	—
10. Rocking Chair	—	20	—	—	—

Exercise Session#:	Repetitions per Session				
	51	52	53	54	55
12. Hand-and-Toe Sit-Up	40	—	42	44	45
13. Cherry Picker	20	20	20	20	20
14. Back Flutter Kick	350	—	360	365	370
15. Stomach Flutter Kick	—	—	120	125	—
16. Sitting Flutter Kick	—	170	175	180	125
17. Back Roller	12	—	—	—	—
18. Stomach Stretcher	—	38	40	41	35
19. Sitting Knee Bend	20	—	—	—	—
20. Leg Lever	—	—	—	—	20
21. Leg Thrust	—	30	—	—	—
22. Legs Flexing, Shoulders Secured	12	—	12	12	12
23. Back Flexing, Legs Secured	12	—	12	12	12
24. Side Flexing, Legs Secured	12	—	12	12	12
25. Sitting Back Bends	12	12	12	12	—
27. Deep Knee Bender, Four-Count	30	30	—	—	30
28. Deep Knee Bender, Two-Count	—	35	—	—	40
30. Leg Stretcher	12	12	12	12	10
31. Thigh Stretcher	12	12	12	12	12
32. Groin Stretcher, Four-Count	—	14	—	14	—
33. Groin Stretcher, Two-Count	—	14	—	14	—
35. One-Legged Sit-Up	—	12	—	12	—
36. Bend and Reach	—	—	12	—	—
40. Deep Breather	6	—	6	—	6
41. Eight-Count Body Builder	22	—	22	—	24
43. One-Legged Push-Up	—	50	—	50	—
44. Press Press Fling	12	12	12	12	12
45. Up Back and Over	12	12	12	12	12
46. Pull-Up	8	8	8	8	8

Week 11:
Running Schedule

	Minutes per Hike				
Hike#:	51	52	53	54	55
Run/Sprint	25	25	25	25	25
Walk	5	5	5	5	5
Run/Sprint	20	20	20	20	20
Walk	10	10	10	10	10
Total Run Time	45	45	45	45	45
Total Walk Time	15	15	15	15	15

Comments

- You may wish to start thinking about things you can do to maintain a superior level of conditioning after completing this program. If you will be playing a sport on a regular basis, this may not be a consideration. If you won't be playing a sport on a regular basis, consider signing up for some 10k road races. They can serve as an excellent incentive to keep yourself in training.

Week 12:
Calisthenics Schedule

	Repetitions per Session				
Exercise Session#:	56	57	58	59	60
1. Full Jumping Jack	50	50	50	50	50
2. Half Jumping Jack	—	20	20	20	20
3. Side Twister Stretcher	—	—	20	20	—
4. Trunk Rotation	16	16	—	—	16
5. Trunk Bending Fore and Aft	—	20	20	20	20
6. Trunk Twister	20	20	20	20	20
7. Windmill, Four-Count	—	20	20	20	20

	Repetitions per Session				
Exercise Session#:	56	57	58	59	60
8.. Windmill, Two-Count	—	35	26	26	20
9. Trunk Side Stretcher	20	20	20	20	20
10. Rocking Chair	20	—	—	—	—
11. Regulation Sit-Up	50	—	—	—	—
12. Hand-and-Toe Sit-Up	—	48	—	—	50
13. Cherry Picker	20	20	—	—	10
14. Back Flutter Kick	—	350	375	375	400
15. Stomach Flutter Kick	—	130	135	135	—
16. Sitting Flutter Kick	125	—	—	—	—
17. Back Roller	—	10	—	—	10
18. Stomach Stretcher	35	—	—	—	50
20. Leg Lever	20	—	—	—	—
21. Leg Thrust	—	—	35	35	—
22. Legs Flexing, Shoulders Secured	12	12	—	—	—
23. Back Flexing, Legs Secured	12	12	—	—	—
24. Side Flexing, Legs Secured	12	12	—	—	—
25. Sitting Back Bends	12	—	—	12	12
27. Deep Knee Bender, Four-Count	—	30	30	30	—
28. Deep Knee Bender, Two-Count	—	40	35	35	—
30. Leg Stretcher	12	12	12	12	12
31. Thigh Stretcher	12	15	12	12	12
32. Groin Stretcher, Four-Count	—	—	16	16	16
33. Groin Stretcher, Two-Count	—	—	16	16	16
34. Calf Stretcher	—	15	20	20	—
37. Squat Stretch	—	—	—	8	—
38. Good Morning Darling	32	—	—	—	—
40. Deep Breather	—	6	—	6	—
41. Eight-Count Body Builder	—	24	—	24	25
43. One-Legged Push-Up	52	—	54	54	—
44. Press Press Fling	12	12	12	12	12
45. Up Back and Over	12	12	12	12	12
46. Pull-Up	8	8	9	9	10

Week 12:
Running Schedule

Hike#:	56	57	58	59	60
			Minutes per Hike		
Run/Sprint	25	25	25	25	25
Walk	5	5	5	5	5
Run/Spring	20	20	20	20	20
Walk	10	10	10	10	10
Total Run Time	45	45	45	45	45
Total Walk Time	15	15	15	15	15

Comments

- At the end of this week, have someone take an "after" picture of you wearing exactly what you were wearing for your "before" picture. Then compare the two pictures. For me, the difference was so dramatic I knew I could *never* go back—and I never did.
- Take your at-rest pulse rate and compare it to the reading you recorded during Week 0. I'm told that by keeping my own pulse rate at about fifty-eight beats per minute, I could be adding several years onto my life expectancy.
- Here are some further maintenance suggestions: After Week 12, continue an exercise regimen by alternately performing the calisthenics schedules for Weeks 4 and 5; and continue running by following the schedule for Hikes 21–60 three times a week (every other day). Don't try to do too much; do only what *you know* you won't back away from (to probably nothing at all) after the intoxication of success has subsided.
- Don't forget to indulge yourself with that special reward you promised yourself. You deserve it!

Author's Note

If you would like to be added to the roll of men and women who have successfully completed this program, please send your name and address to me, in care of the publisher (the address is on the copyright page). Include both the date you started the program and the date you completed it. Also, if you wish, include a few words about your experience with the program, and about any changes the program may have brought about in your life. You may also wish to include a copy of your Personal Record.

Personal Record

Keeping statistics can be a good way of demonstrating progress and therefore of keeping your morale up. Hence, you may wish to use the following chart to keep a weekly record of your weight, waist or hip size, biceps, thighs, and pulse rate (both at-rest and active). To ensure accuracy, take all measurements at the same time of day, beginning with the end of Week 0.

You can also use this chart to keep a count of the total number of miles you have run. You will need to estimate your mileage figures, however, because the Running Program is structured in minutes rather than miles. If you run the same few routes, you may be able to measure the distances involved with the odometer on a car; if not, use a pedometer, properly calibrated to your pace. (If you use a pedometer, you may wish to walk off the distances, to ensure a consistent pace.)

Personal Record Chart

Start Date _____

End of:	Weight	Waist/Hips	Biceps	Thighs
Week 0	_____	_____	_____	_____
Week 1	_____	_____	_____	_____
Week 2	_____	_____	_____	_____
Week 3	_____	_____	_____	_____
Week 4	_____	_____	_____	_____
Week 5	_____	_____	_____	_____
Week 6	_____	_____	_____	_____
Week 7	_____	_____	_____	_____
Week 8	_____	_____	_____	_____
Week 9	_____	_____	_____	_____
Week 10	_____	_____	_____	_____
Week 11	_____	_____	_____	_____
Week 12	_____	_____	_____	_____

End Date _____

End of:	Pulse (at rest)	Pulse (after sprint)	Miles This Week	Total Miles
Week 0				
Week 1				
Week 2				
Week 3				
Week 4				
Week 5				
Week 6				
Week 7				
Week 8				
Week 9				
Week 10				
Week 11				
Week 12